Eating Myself

CANDIDA CREWE

BLOOMSBURY

First published 2006
This paperback edition published 2007

Copyright © 2006 by Candida Crewe

The moral right of the author has been asserted

Bloomsbury Publishing Plc
36 Soho Square
London W1D 3QY

A CIP catalogue record for this book
is available from the British Library

ISBN 9780747585626

10 9 8 7 6 5 4 3 2 1

Typeset by Hewer Text UK Ltd, Edinburgh
Printed by Clays Ltd, St Ives plc

All papers used by Bloomsbury Publishing are natural,
recyclable products made from wood grown in well-managed
forests. The manufacturing processes conform to the
environmental regulations of the country of origin.

www.bloomsbury.com/candidacrewe

For Mama

Alarm Clock

I am five-foot five and three quarters. My weight over the years has been as follows:

From the age of eighteen to twenty-three, a steady 10 stone 5 lbs.

Following eleven-week starvation diet aged twenty three, 7 stone 13 lbs.

The bulimia years, aged twenty-three to twenty-eight or twenty-nine, 9 stone 2 lbs to 11 stone 3 lbs (my heaviest ever).

My wedding, 4th January 1997, aged thirty-two, 9 stone 4 lbs.

Q Trust dinner, 2nd February 2004, aged thirty-nine, 8 stone 10 lbs.

Current average, aged forty, between 8 stone 12 lbs and 9 stone 4 lbs.

Following pneumonia, Christmas 2005, 8 stone 7 lbs.

Yesterday, 8 February 2005, 8 stone 12 lbs.

Today, 9 February 2005, 8 stone 13 lbs.

Tomorrow?

Breakfast

For three days, I tasted peanut-butter pizza, peanut-butter omelette, peanut-butter pie, peanut-butter punch and peanut-butter ice cream. In fact, just about every unreasonable manifestation of peanut butter you can imagine.

I was in Orlando, Florida, staying at a big, modern hotel, marble interior, foyer as glazed and soft as a tinned peach. The centenary convention of the Adults Only Peanut Butter Lovers' Fan Club was being held there. I was not a member. I was writing about it. I quite like crunchy peanut butter and have been known to dig into a jar for a clot of it so as to gulp it off the end of my finger. I'm not one averse to that slight gag on the roof of the mouth, of fine mud granules in carpet pile. But I'm not like committed member Jeanie Character, who had to have her stomach stapled in Gainesville because she and peanut butter were like *that*.

When it was all over and I was on the plane to New York, I was wearing a beloved viscose skirt because, if I felt full, it flowed freely. It had an elastic waistband which created a fleshy frieze round me of conceptual etchings in pink, but was not so tight that it challenged my breathing. It was loose round my thighs and, on balance, afforded an impression of security. I hadn't overeaten but hadn't exactly been the paragon of restraint either; I'd tried plenty of those cloying

3

recipes. The majority of – mostly American – peanut butter fans, some who had driven 3,000 miles so as not to miss the convention, were eye-poppingly fat. It was as if only their eyes were holding them up inside this outsize costume, their feet dangling out of view somewhere round the knees. I wanted to step up on a stool, look into their mouths, hold my hand out to them. I knew it was dark in there.

These people made me like and respect them. Publicly, at least, they were not bowed. I realised there is my kind of fat, and fat. Their size was of a different order. It had the advantage of allowing me to put a spoonful of food into my mouth, to sample some of the peanut butter offerings, without the usual need to flinch from dumb eyes judging. I was grateful to them for that.

My shoulder was pressed against the panel beside the cardboard door of the aeroplane lavatory. The wallpaper, surface texture of porridge, was cream with faint grey pictures of spitfires and clouds. I was troubling them with my forefinger. And glancing every few seconds at the little light-up red man, but he was obstinate in his occupied slot.

'I apologise, Madam, have you been waiting long?' Concerned voice.

The air hostess, with her firm blue uniform, mannered bun and compulsory figure, looked at my stomach.

It is faces that have histories, or so they say. People talk of old ladies made beautiful by laughter lines, a rather sentimental misconception but a compelling one nonetheless. We like to think it is the face, window to the soul and all that, which tells the story, and though the story's rarely laughter, it comforts us to think so. But it's not necessarily even heartbreak and regret that fashions the face. That is a romantic notion. It is years of moaning and coffee, paperwork and sun, reading in poor light and spilt milk. My face certainly has more prosaic tell-tales than crinkles created of heady hilarity, grand passions untimely ripped and spiritual enlightenment. Above my lip there is a faint, faint scar, from a fall through a floorboard aged three. There is another one, equally undramatic, beside my right eye: a car crash on the way back from a dancing lesson when I was four. A pale pink blemish on my left cheek: shadow of a spot I picked as a teenager, less forgiving than all the rest, the one which chose to serve me right. So what? No, I don't think my face has much to tell. My stomach on the other hand . . . My stomach's the place to look for my history. And though it has never seen the light of day – I don't want people to look at it even as it is, perennially covered in capacious layers – it is the thing which shaped me.

I traced the journey of the air hostess's eyes, and when they landed, flies on shit, I tensed.

Then her punch-line. 'Are you pregnant?'

A year or so ago, when my third and last child was nine months old, I took my middle son to tea with a little boy he had met in the park. His mother had also invited some of her friends and their children to join us. One, with a toddler and a neat bump, told me she was a writer. She wanted to impress upon me how good she was, but tedious restraints of social convention dictated she could not. So instead she bloomed at me. Her bloom was with the pride and pleasure of being a writer and being six months pregnant. But, even more, it was the bloom of being six months pregnant and only looking three.

She took in my stomach. Then, breezy voice: 'Are you having another?'

*   *   *

5

A few weeks ago my cousin told me about a foolish man. He was called David. She had met him at the house of some colleagues. Another guest was a woman in her thirties who was there with her husband. David congratulated her on her news.

'You haven't found out the sex, have you?' he asked eagerly.

The woman frowned.

'I'm telling you, it's a boy,' he enthused, 'and, what's more, I'm always right. A boy it is. How exciting! No, don't look so surprised. You thought it was a girl, didn't you? Look, we'll do the test.'

Without further ado he slipped off his wedding ring, tied it on a piece of string and dangled it over the woman's stomach. It swung the boy way.

'You see! I was right. It *is* a boy.' Pause. 'But you don't look too pleased. You wanted a girl? Don't worry, I've got two boys, and they're great. Anyway, next time . . .'

'I'm not pregnant.'

When my cousin told me that story, I quivered with that woman's humiliation, for it might as well have been my own. I have never forgotten the post-peanut butter incident on the aeroplane, although it took place fifteen years ago; and since that children's tea, I have not been able to bring myself to invite back, even ring, the amiable mother who hosted it because I don't want to be reminded of her blooming friend. I expect there are some – not many – women who can shrug and laugh when they are mistaken for pregnant. My hat goes off. I am not one of them.

My fear of being fat is no longer morbid, but it is dogged enough that the man or woman who comments on my size, erroneously takes my swollen belly for happy fecundity, is neither forgotten nor forgiven.

In my early twenties I spun away into the realms of a gruesome eating disorder and my daydreams glinted with images of blades slicing away flesh from my stomach and hips and thighs. The knives have since been put away, and my dysfunction around food is now normal in as much as, while it may have a more extreme history, it doesn't wildly differ from that of every woman I have known or have ever met.

My survey would not impress the men from Mori; it is an inexact science, bred of serious, casual and overheard conversations, of the heightened observation of a figure obsessed by her subject. I am constantly on the alert, ears ever pricked for the signs. I see them all the time; it is like learning a new word and hearing it for ever after. I don't think I'm particularly peculiar but these signs are all about me. I do not claim to have known or met an inordinate amount of people, to have travelled to the ends of the earth and exhaustively interviewed women of different ages and cultures on the subject. But I read newspapers and books, go to the cinema, watch television, listen to the radio, and everywhere I do go – be it to the local supermarket checkout, a social gathering, the school steps, a bar, an airport in a far-off land, an unknown city in a foreign country, up a mountain, anywhere – I am listening to women who speak of diets, feeling fat, loathing their very flesh; who voice consummate anxiety at not being thin, even if they are. It is a female language which, from my heightened perspective, is seemingly spoken by every woman, from a fish-finger factory worker in Grimsby to an au pair brought up in a remote village of the Czech Republic, to a grandmother from Grenada. Some speak it more fluently than others, but I have never come across a woman who hasn't understood it to some degree, and had at least some grasp of its basic structure and vocabulary. Even those few who don't have much use for it – in forty years, I have met just a handful – if they have any girlfriends at all, or enjoy the company of other women, they hear it all the time so are able to understand it. It is the continuous female soundtrack, silent as well as spoken, of guilt and anxiety. Voiced, it turns into a kind of sisterly shorthand, one which by its very nature is appealing for collusion, acknowledgement, recognition, reassurance, solace and support. 'I mustn't.' 'Oh, go on then.' 'I will if you will.' 'Will someone share it with me?' 'I'll be good, starting tomorrow.' It is a given that any food more evolved than a leaf is pushing it; any food with a whiff of fat or sugar about it a kind of insanity. Giving into it simply cannot be done with the all-male silent gusto with which a man sets about a king-size Mars bar, a tabloid of chips or a sticky toffee pudding. Women will not do it without some kind of nod to the greed of it. It must always be justified. It's a one-off madness, a rare loss of control with a symbiotic excuse: 'I haven't stopped or sat down all day, I think I deserve a treat.' 'It's Sally's birthday.' 'It's Christmas next week.' 'My cat just died.' This language even has a signing version. Tapping a stomach with a flattened palm means, thanks, no more, got to be careful. Forefinger pointing downwards into the cake mixture says, I mean to have this much, just tasting, and then stop. This is my native language. I've studied it with passion all along, and I'm saying the abnormal is normal and the extremes – namely anorexia, bulimia and compulsive over-eating – no longer really extremes, just a variant of that all-too normal.

*   *   *

In 1993, I went to stay a night with the Anglo-Irish novelist, Molly Keane, at her house an hour's drive west of Cork. It was high up with a startling view over a September sea and deserted beach; the garden was full of fuchsia bushes, their flowers as plump as dancing crinolines. On the sofa in her small sitting-room, Molly looked frail. She was nearly ninety and just six stone. Her old tweed skirt was loose, thin lilac pop socks and a lukewarm hot-water bottle her meagre defences against the cold. We talked into the waning afternoon.

Dinner that night, just the two of us, was an expansive affair. We had home-made soup to start with, followed by roast chicken, gravy, bread sauce, roast potatoes and parsnips, sprouts and carrots. Next, Queen of Puddings, a fabulous concoction of meringue, custard and strawberry jam eaten with Blyton lashings of cream. Molly, not letting me get up from my chair, shuffled to the sideboard and plunged a silver tablespoon into the pudding's sugary tulle.

'How much would you like, my darling?' she asked.

'Very little, please,' I said dutifully, calorie costs ringing up loudly and tiresomely inside my head. My instinct was not to have any at all because Queen of Puddings was beyond the pale, so much so as barely to merit temptation. I had myself well-trained. And yet this had been cooked specially for my visit; I could hardly picture Molly, left to her own devices, surviving on anything more substantial than a little light consommé. So it was that manners towards an old lady for once prevailed over the workings of my ever-dieting mind. Even so, very little, please, was the best I could do.

'Why?' she asked.

I patted my stomach by way of explanation. Molly nodded. She knew exactly what I meant. But then, ever mischievous and generous, she ignored me and carried on spooning the pudding on to my plate.

'Ah well,' I said, giving in; no choice. I was inwardly panicking and trying to justify to myself accepting such a large helping. 'Donovan has said he would still love me even if I were eighteen stone.'

Molly immediately stopped serving and put the spoon down. She handed me the plate.

'Ah, yes, my darling,' she said, knowing, 'but if I were you, I wouldn't risk it.'

My normal abnormality is that I think about food or weight on average every few seconds.

It is a constant with me, on the brain, same as they say sex is for men. From the moment I wake up in the morning I think about it. In those five more minutes before that final push out of bed, I am not relishing the last sleep-sozzled moments of peace like most people; instead the mind is already racing apace with fat-related questions. I ask myself, lying there, covered in blankets and husband asleep and unaware, no one in the world to see me, not even myself, does it matter *at this precise moment* that I am fat? It doesn't, strictly, I say to myself, the mattering is only in the anticipation of getting up and out of bed and becoming part of the world and being visible again. I wonder that I cannot cast aside the anticipation, just for a little bit, the five minutes between waking and rising, and enjoy the feelings of release they could bestow if only I knew how to let them. I stabilise myself with one thought before I get out of bed. Not, is it Tuesday, but, how fat am I today? Wouldn't it be nice if I were to awaken one morning and find I was miraculously thin. Foolish fantasy instantly sidelined by reality. So what is it actually to be? A Very Fat, Fat, or Marginally Less Fat day?

The answer, which depends on a kaleidoscope of factors, is instantaneous because those factors are so very well established even in my groggy, waking mind that there is no room for confusion. They include a computer-quick till receipt of the complete intake of food over the previous two to three days, down to the last grape, a hand's rummage, surgical in its expertise, over the trifle surface of the naked stomach to assess it in all that particular morning's imperfections (its curvature: quite how acute?), then I note if that familiar feeling of ickiness, which a friend has called 'clarty', is present or absent. Clarty can be just a hangover from too much garlic the night before, or too much food, full stop, the whole of the previous day or days. It is a feeling, a degree off nausea, which lurks, possibly in the throat, although its location is indistinct, and the physical sensation of it has the clever knock-on effect of pressing on the psychological. Clarty makes me feel fat. The days it is there can never be Marginally Less Fat days. Clarty days are invariably Very Fat days, but there can also be Very Fat days without a trace of clarty. Up for consideration next, before I'll stick a foot out of bed, is exactly how heavy I am. I might be in weighing mode, in which case I can leap up, go for a crucial pee (for the sake of economy). Naked, adrenaline kicking in, I step on the scales and discover what my mood is to be for the day. Or maybe it's a period when I'm not allowing myself the scales crutch, in which case I make a wild guess anyway and my mood alters accordingly, just as if I'd seen the read-out after all. Now that I have digital scales, I have the dubious luxury of being able to measure myself – or not, as the case may be – in ounces as well as stones and pounds. (I was born in the

Sixties. While I can do kilograms, they are still something of a foreign language; I can't quite gauge their *feel*.) Once my mood was cast low by a pound gained or elevated by a pound lost. It is now with the measly ounce that its sheep-like destiny lies.

All things taken into account, while still in bed or just out of it, how confident am I allowed to be today? Lying there, I remind myself I never want ideas above my confidence station. This is run entirely according to my weight; the tighter the ship, the greater the confidence. This means that on a Very Fat day, I can only wear black and not be too noisy or noticeable, must keep my eyes cast down to the ground; on a merely Fat day, I can wear any colour as long as it is black and can talk quietly if I keep my eyes to myself. On a Marginally Less Fat day, colour can creep in, if only muted browns and greys, and then only on my upper body, and I can make someone laugh as long as I do so quickly. I can even stick up for myself and make a sharp remark, fashionably *assert* myself, mildly. But it's a risk I rarely take.

If I had been a thin person I think I would have been a bitch.

As I see it, ludicrously, it's all right to be a bitch if you're not fat. There's the physical superiority which guarantees you licence to get away with it. I don't argue with thin people. Going to the park, three children in the back of the car, I had a stand-off with a woman in a fat Jeep. She wouldn't reverse to let me pass, and nor would I. Road-rage raring, I got out and approached her window – this story does not reflect well on me – and told her she had my sympathy, she must be an unhappy type, *not to go back three bloody feet* just because she was *under the mistaken impression* she got there first. Through the self-important smokiness of her window, I could detect her lips sphincter. She wouldn't look at me, she wouldn't budge. Toddler-like, I stomped back to my car – head-to-head with hers, bumpers almost necking – and switched off my engine. I'm like that. It's hardly attractive, but I'm not averse to a bit of confrontation when I think I'm in the right and it's not a Very Fat day. Had it been one of those, I would not have got myself into that position in the first place. I would have reversed at the outset and kissed her arse. But it just so happened that that day was a Marginally Thinner day, so I had more confidence at my disposal. I stayed behind the wheel, prepared for a long sit-in. Three minutes later she crashed out of her door and marched up to me. She'd given in first. I was triumphant. But not so fast. She was my age, with the thick, textured complexion of a shop mannequin and expensive hair. There was an air about her of someone who was recently divorced, a certain bitter vengefulness which a brush with the family courts can perfect in a person. My face was naked and my hair, which has been described as beach, was at its beachiest. I was wearing a cheap coat with give-away fake fur trim, matted, around the hood. White trash in my white Vauxhall. She told me she wasn't surprised I wasn't going to back up because, she shouted, I looked 'like a *feminist*'. She really let herself down at that moment, but it was short-lived, my sense of triumph. I watched her raging at me, didn't hear another word she said and couldn't deliver any of my own. All I could see was that she had on cream jeans, an item of clothing as far from my ken as a chain-mail doublet, and legs up to her nostrils. The comedy of her insult had not passed me by. She was stupider than me but she was thinner. Because I was fatter than her, I could say nothing. Fat and a bitch makes you a fat bitch. I was proud of 'feminist', but I couldn't risk 'fat bitch'. In my book, insults don't come much more reductive. Lowest of the low. You might as well dig yourself into a hole and stay there.

I am not saying that all thin women are bitches but thin women do have that choice. Of course fat women do too and there are plenty who are every bit as spoilt, thoughtless, selfish, mean-spirited and unkind as some thin women. It is just that I don't acknowledge them in my mind because my mind is full of the stereotype – the rounded, jolly fat person whose sense of humour, whose sweetness and warmth, diverts attention from or makes up for a physical shape that does not fit the ideal mould. For years I have read interviews with people who were fat as children and claimed that the way they deflected potential bullies was by making them laugh. I have grown a shameful prejudice which means I am mostly blind to the bitchy side of fat people. A sort of inverted fatism results in my overlooking their traits and only seeing the best in them. When I was myself, briefly, thinner, I did not become a bitch because I had been fat for far too long and knew my place. I still thought like a fat person and was heavily aware that I was probably not going to manage to stay 'thin' for more than a matter of days or weeks. God forbid that I should settle into my new skin too complacently, adapt my nature too radically to fit my new body type. That way, when weight started to reappear, any popularity I might have gained would plummet. I would be a write-off.

So it is, with the morning checklist complete – the kind of day acknowledged, and clothes and confidence allowance established (in collaboration with my historical context, naturally) – I can walk downstairs and finally contemplate what is in store for me, over the next twelve hours or so, in terms of food. Rarely specifics at this early stage of the morning but projected volumes permissible in the course of the day ahead – minimal, normal or lots. The quantities of each are clear in my mind though they invariably differ from other people's definitions. If the answer is minimal, then I feel both slightly depressed at the proposed deprivation but consoled at its possible effect. Normal feels OK, but I can't be doing with that every day, it smacks too much of boring moderation. Filling is good – the anticipated pleasure of satisfying food and a satisfied stomach – and bad, namely the potential resulting roll.

As I lay out cereal bowls for the children and shake some Shreddies into them, my mind turns to breakfast, mildly. I don't think about eating it much. I'm past that. But as I watch them chomping away at their third piece of toast, either grumpily or cheerfully depending on their night, and my husband being willingly assaulted by a full cafetière of real coffee and the occasional Ulster Fry, I ponder upon people who never eat breakfast.

You know those people who don't eat breakfast. 'I don't eat breakfast,' they say and the tone they use has in it, if you listen carefully, little orange flecks of pride. 'Just a cup of black coffee and a fag,' they say, and that makes them superior to you.

I am one of those people who does eat breakfast. There is a saying about smokers which maintains that people fall into four categories. There are smokers who smoke, smokers who don't smoke, non-smokers who smoke (I was one of them when I was trying in my late teens and twenties to redeem some kind of cool to make up for being a fat, square, non-drinking sad fuck) and non-smokers who don't smoke (which is what I am now and have been ever since I realised at thirty that my original category really was untenably foolish). It is the same with breakfasters (the breakfasting breakfasters among them, as far as I can make out, an endangered species). I am someone who by nature very much eats breakfast but who doesn't, if you see what I mean. Through sheer force of will I have trained myself, congenital breakfaster that I am, never to go anywhere near it.

I have tremendous memories of many years enjoying what anyone will tell me is the most important meal of the day. (My mother hates the word 'meal' – 'hot meal' really gets her down – as she has a very visual mind and it conjures up for her pictures of chicken or rabbit feed, and she never used to let me use it. I hear where she is coming from, but it can be quite useful so I make no apologies.) Her special porridge looms large in amongst these memories, as well as bowls of Frosties glistening in cold and creamy milk, brown-speckled boiled eggs and soldiers with melting butter, toasted home-made bread with more melting butter and home-made High Dumpsy Deary jam courtesy of a woman in Marlborough called Edith who had a whole wondrous shop just full of her chutneys and preserves. These breakfasts were something which, when I was at boarding-school, I looked forward to for weeks between exeats. Mum would come to pick up me and a friend early on a Sunday morning, we would drive twenty minutes across the frosty downs and arrive back at the cottage for a breakfast extravaganza.

But then sometime in my teens, during the four desultory years at my school in Oxford when friends were discovering the – laxative? – joys of early morning caffeine and cigarettes, breakfast became uncool. The most this dubious version of cool would allow was 'a quick slice of toast' but even that was considered de trop. Giving up breakfast began to make sense. In one stroke it would mean that I would turn into one of those noble souls who was above such things and at the same time lop a third off the day's calorie intake. When, aged eighteen, I finally moved back to London, city of my birth and youth and right and uncertain happiness, I had successfully transformed myself into one of those people who never eats breakfast and I have regretfully remained one of them ever since.

I say regretfully because, although a habit of over twenty years means that I am never hungry in the mornings any more, the truth is, I love breakfast. I miss the idea of it very much. On those rare occasions when I am staying in a hotel I see it displayed in the middle of whispering dining rooms, a kind of wanton come-on to even the most breakfast-chaste souls such as myself. There is freshly squeezed orange juice; there is Greek yoghurt and honey; there are dried fruits; brioches and plain, almond and chocolate croissants, Danish pastries and toast, warm rolls; mueslis of various complexions, cornflakes; sausages, bacon, rich, yellow, fried and scrambled eggs, and that eighth deadly sin, one of my favourite foods of yesteryear, black pudding. I watch my fellow guests dithering with joy at the sheer choice and temptation before them and giving in to it, rapturously. I stare at their nonchalance and abandon in wonder. So, I think to myself, coffee-and-fag brigade be damned, there are plenty of happy breakfasting breakfasters after all. But perhaps only in hotels. Perhaps these people are non-breakfasters who are breakfasting just because they are in a hotel and would not do so normally. Who knows. There again, people, friends, are beginning to talk about breakfast once more, buying Cheerios and making boiled eggs for their children, grabbing a croissant and a full-on cappuccino on their way to work. One woman I know makes her own muesli and it is inspired. Clare and Jan both say, quite openly, 'God, how can you not eat breakfast? I'd faint before ten!' How indeed? I am no longer a slave to the urge to be cool (age, motherhood, general resignation); I would like to eat breakfast again. The trouble is, after all this time, not eating it has become part of my system, so deep-rooted now that to go back to my natural, breakfasting self would be unspeakably hard. I have lost the wherewithal. It is not a question of just leaping out of bed tomorrow morning and saying, right, make that a bowl of Grape Nuts and two slices of toast with marmalade for me. In breakfast's place, for the past fifteen years or so, I have put my daily fix of a tablespoon of linseeds which I swallow – never chew, that would be eating – teaspoon by teaspoon with a pint glass of water to make the medicine go down. These seeds are not strictly medicine; you buy them in boxes in healthfood shops, and they are a dead ringer for Trill and a natural remedy for constipation. After my bouts of anorexia and bulimia and their concomitant gridlock of the digestive system, I became a sucker for the most expensive brand, Linusit Gold, or Linushit Gold, as Char's husband, James, calls it, and have been dependent ever since. Taken with liquid these shiny seeds swell a little in the gut and become all mucusy. This helps everything to flow along with the happy ease of mild liquid handwash through the dispenser in a public lavatory. I know that since taking up this linseed habit I have kept off weight that would otherwise have clung about me unhealthily. They are one of the main reasons why I am consistently a stone and five pounds lighter than I was throughout my late teens and early twenties. Or so I like to believe. Whatever, there is not a morning that passes without my gulping them down. The packet recommends you tart them up a bit with fruit juice or yoghurt or the cereal of your choice, but that would feel like sailing a bit close to the breakfast wind. Water, calories 0, does for me.

It may be less interesting but it's better than coffee. I don't drink coffee, partly because if I did I would probably take it with sugar and milk. Coffee: great smell, just can't stand the taste (though translated into cake or ice cream I can stand it all too well). Nor tea. The only hot drinks I like are hot chocolate and – it is taking quite a lot out of me to admit this bearing in mind I've a while to go yet before I collect my pension – Horlicks. A three-course lunch in a mug! Forget it. My system states that both are off limits so I never touch either. What I drink without fail every morning an hour or so after my intake of bird feed is a 330 ml can of carbonated water, colour (E150d), flavourings (including caffeine), sweeteners (aspartame, acesulfame K), phosphoric acid, citric acid, preservative (E211) and a source of phenylalanine. It is an unholy mixture and the aspartame in it apparently triggers migraines, kills brain cells and causes extensive nerve damage, as well as promoting depression, tumours and cancers. Otherwise identified as Diet Coke, it weighs in at a marvellous 0.4 kcal per 100 ml and it has been a habit of mine since shortly after the filthy stuff was introduced to the world in 1982.

I had never been much of a Coca-Cola fiend. A voluptuous glass bottle of it, while it had certain charm on a hot, hot day, seemed to represent an awful lot of calories for not very much return. (It gave rise only to fleeting abdominal satisfaction compared to that following a packet of cheese straws, say, or a brace of jam doughnuts.) I could live without it. But when its diet counterpart hit the general consciousness, with its alluring promise of just one calorie per can, what woman like me could resist? (Diet Pepsi, own-brand colas, and, God forbid, syrup-fizzy-water-mix colas from taps in cinemas and pubs, will never do.) Christina Onassis, the heiress who long struggled with her weight, was said, when she died aged thirty-seven following years of drug abuse, to have had a serious Diet Coke habit to boot. Reports in the papers at the time – it was 1988 – stated that she regularly had consignments of the stuff delivered to her home(s). The news did give pause. I am not sure why as it wasn't the Diet Coke which had seen her off, and the Nutrasweet (aspartame) scares had not at that stage hit (my) home. But I was on a two-litre bottle a day and I knew it couldn't be good. This was a drink that actually tasted of something but was only a fraction more expensive (in the calorie economy) than water. It was a drink for free. Of course I knew fine well, really, that you don't get anything for nothing, that with every sip I was edging closer to something catastrophic at the hands of its unknown, almost certainly sinister properties. But women everywhere took it to their bosoms – especially fat ones like me and Christina Onassis. Diet Coke appeals to us more than to men, even if its marketing boys would not have it thus. As a general rule, men spurn it as they spurn quiche or fresh fruit; they still prefer the meat and three veg version. (I have encountered grown men who, if they take a swig of mine by mistake, do the nose trick and make dramatic noises.) I only know one woman who drinks classic as opposed to Diet Coke and that's my friend Sophie. But Sophie has fat-defying legs and tends to have a rather masculine way about her at times so she doesn't count.

Over twenty years on – oh, God, is it that much? Well, it is bound to be the ruin of me – I have cut back to my one can a day. Times I try to give it up completely. What I am doing to my brain cells periodically seizes my imagination. I see them like the numerous little soldiers in my son's detailed drawings, being decimated by the slings and arrows of aspartame and the fearful forces of formaldehyde (aspartame's by-product and closest ally). Their collective destruction means I myself am heading for certain premature senility and possible horrible death. I stop buying my multipack cans for a few days, then spot on the shelves the new with-a-twist-of-lemon spin and am tempted to try it. It tastes like the chemical citrus smell of those tree-shaped air fresheners which swing from the windscreen mirrors in dodgy minicabs. Can we really not bother to slice a real, live lemon any more? I am not falling for that one. But then an over-sweet but lovely vanilla version appears on the market. Vanilla is my favourite smell and taste. When labels on vanilla shower gels and body milks say THIS IS NOT FOOD, I see the point. I could live on vanilla. I recently read a whole book about the stuff. (It mentioned that the embrace by Coca-Cola of this precious ingredient has been making ripples anew in a trade that has always been delicate and rivals that of cocaine for cartels, intrigue and mysterious deaths.) Of course vanilla Diet Coke has my name all over it. I try it and am hooked once more.

There has been talk on the Net recently that, quite apart from despatching habitual drinkers to their early demise, Diet Coke isn't even diet. Artificial sweeteners apparently trick the body so it thinks and behaves as if they were real sugars anyway and starts craving more carbohydrate. I can't quite believe that. Or don't want to. My cynical old body is surely not so easily fooled. As I tuck into my non-breakfast can – on an empty stomach and sometimes as early as eight in the morning; it is a habit which makes a dawn cigarette seem like a health choice – I console myself with this thought: if all the Diet Coke I have ever drunk had been real Coke I would not have a tooth in my head by now and, more tragically, I would have become the size of a six-bedroom house. I can live with the thought of dementia.

I clear the children's detritus away. There are always soggy bits of Special K lurking in dregs of milk like discarded gloves in a puddle and crusts of toast with smudges of butter and jam, but I do not pick. I don't even think of it as food, see it merely as mess to be binned but not into me. I have learned to shelve hunger in the morning and cannot begin to contemplate food in any detail until later. After breakfast, theirs not mine, I can go shopping for the ingredients for lunch and supper but while doing so separate myself from thoughts of actually eating it, divorce desires. Those, I reckon, must wait.

So, anyway, that's breakfast.

Most days, most seconds, I reckon that between seven to fourteen pounds would do the trick. If I could lose that amount of weight and keep it off without too much of a feeling of deprivation, I would, I believe, at last be content.

Fifty per cent of women in the UK are on a diet at any one time. Seventy per cent have been on one and, though there is no statistic I know of to prove it, you can bet most of the remaining lot have thought about dieting even if they haven't ever quite got round to it. There is an assumption that the women most exercised by their weight are those from the upper and middle classes because, the argument goes, they can afford the luxury of such neuroses and expensive, fresh food that is not as fattening as cheap, processed pap. Indeed figures reveal that those from lower-income families are the ones more prone to obesity. That may be the case but that does not mean they care about it less. We are continually exposed to a media obsessed with emaciation, to pictures of stringy celebrities who, though they have little or no fat, appear to have it all, and the drip-drip effect reaches everyone.

It is wrong to say that those who allow themselves to become fat are uneducated and do not care. Obesity and its attendant dangers are in the news. Education about health and exercise is in the news. There are popular television series devoted to the subject and diet books sell by the million. You would have to be a hermit not to know that five – a figure which recently increased to nine – portions of fruit and vegetables a day are good, McDonald's hamburgers and chips bad. Such information, and its resulting concerns, are not the preserve of a chattering elite who have nothing better to do than spend all day in exclusive gyms, pick at rocket salads with their girlfriends in smart restaurants, chew over the maxim that there is no such thing as too rich or too thin and generally contemplate their own navels.

There was a survey in a magazine which said most women would prefer to lose a stone than fall in love or win a million pounds. In a recent poll, fifty-two per cent of American women went so far as to admit that they would give up a year of their lives to stay at an ideal weight. Of the ninety per cent of women in the Western world who want to lose weight the majority are like me, wishing to tackle just a few pounds here and there. It is only the clinically obese, after all, who need to shift stones as opposed to pounds for health reasons, and only those whose perceptions have been skewed by anorexia harbour irrational goals to be morbidly underweight. Most of us are labouring with the bit extra which makes the difference merely between normal (the goalposts of which are, happily, diverse and wide but, unhappily for most women, unacceptable) and thin. Almost all women have a relationship with food that is more loaded than the purely functional – memories of baking with our mothers; eating picnics with friends in the sun, or exotic suppers abroad; the smell of bacon before school; the treat of illicit chocolate biscuits at midnight; the loss of appetite after a break-up; the comfort of cakes and custard. Eating disorders are often, though by no means always, caused by negative associations with the body and food combined with negative circumstances – a less than idyllic childhood, a dysfunctional family life, abuse present and past. But the (less extreme) desire of every woman to be thin, its attendant struggles, failures and guilt, are not so easily accounted for. Most people can lay claim to some unhappy experiences to a greater or lesser degree. For a few, these experiences may have an effect on how they view their bodies; for many more, they may not. Women's quest for thinness in the modern Western world, and beyond, is the contemporary collective condition of being female – because of, in spite of, whatever – the diversity of the female experience. It exists. And is here to stay.

In my mind I see all women attached to a vast, colourful spectrum, individuals dotted about it according to the intensity of their behaviour around food and their attitude to weight. Those with eating disorders are at one end and women who are completely indifferent to the whole damn weight business are at the other, merrily dancing atop the crock of gold. Needless to say this golden end is very under-populated because rare is the woman whose indifference is entirely genuine, bred of proper self-respect and confidence and not falsely manufactured out of feelings of defensiveness. All the rest of us reside at various different points across the middle. Some of us are caught in a particular spot and remain there for a long time. Others move about the spectrum according to our circumstances (crudely, the happier we are, the closer to the crock we inch). The way I see it, it was cultural pressures that created the spectrum in the first place and plastered it with Western women (and, increasingly, with women from the developing world), but our exact position on it is down to our individual stories. The cultural causes are well-documented by historians and commentators who are better placed to write about them than me and whose books – I think for example of *Fat Is a Feminist Issue* and *The Beauty Myth* – I have been known to clutch to my bosom while lumbering about between the reds, the yellows, the indigoes and violets. For myself, I feel I know the whys and the wherefores, from traditional female oppression to today's pernicious influence of fashion, media and magazines and what have you. Don't most of us? And long ago I acknowledged my anger at the pointlessness and injustice and waste of it all, of women's lives diverted by such nonsense. I do not dismiss the urgency and ugliness of the causes, and the troubling and profound misery of their effects on women everywhere – the rise of eating disorders and plastic surgery being sinister examples – or the importance of the rallying against. But what concerns me is the day-to-day reality of the normal-abnormal existence in particular, the actuality of its banal struggle. The day-to-day reality which of course arises from the culture we live in but also from our own experiences and lives and unique context within that culture. I want to examine an individual's story for its influence on where it locates us on the spectrum and I suppose my story, which has some things in common with every woman's, is as good a start as any.

*

The bathing suit I am wearing, astonishing orange with blowsy splats of yellow, is a Sixties masterpiece. Where had my mother found such a thing? But more astonishing is the fact that I am wearing it at all. The bathing suit is not an item of clothing with which I have any truck. I have worn one possibly eight times since 1976. What is more, I am dancing in it, dancing, dancing, on the lawn at Wootton. My limbs are undulating with Super 8 abandon to a music other than the de-de-de beat of the old projector. I watch myself and blink. I am three years old. I have a stomach which starts at my sternum and, round as a water melon, curves perfectly to my pubic bone. Someone once told me that the reason a child's stomach is so distended is because their body is not yet big enough for their own liver, the liver being close to its adult self from birth. I don't seem to be aware of my stomach, or if I am I'm not minding it. For a full four minutes I dance to the silent music – 'Lucy in the Sky with Diamonds'? – and then the screen splutters to white with a silhouette storm of dust.

How soon after that dance was it before the self-consciousness about my stomach set in? It can't have been long. I didn't have long. I don't remember that dance; I have no memories from the time before the worries about the way I look took hold and my sense of inferiority bred of being larger than I should began to ingratiate itself and cling to me like a square person at a party.

Wootton was the village in Bedfordshire where I lived from the age of two till five when my parents were still married.

I was born in London in 1964, the only child of my father's second marriage and my mother's first. I should never have been, really, had the prediction by a physician, in 1932, come true. My father, aged six, had started to fall over a great deal for no apparent reason. He was taken by his mother to Harley Street for an assessment. The grand doctor was creepy. My father said he had hard eyes but his hands, feeling his body, felt soft like a woman's. He told my grandmother that Pop had muscular dystrophy and would die when he was about sixteen. He told Pop he would be all right when he reached that age. With typical Edwardian reserve, my grandmother (whom I never met) did not refer to the matter again for many years and, who knows, perhaps because my father did not anticipate an early death, he did not engender one. He lived till he was seventy-two. He had three wives and five children. He wrote several books and, in a series of ingenious wheelchairs, two designed by friends, he travelled over the years all over the shop, from Tokyo to Timbuktu. It was a life little hampered by his disability; he made sure of that.

My grandmother, Annabel Crewe, was born in 1881. The eldest of three daughters of the Marquis of Crewe, she was brought up on the family estate in Cheshire. The house, Crewe Hall, was early seventeenth century but burnt down in 1866 and was rebuilt. Though impressive, it is no beauty. A faintly hideous redbrick pile laced on the inside with ornate bannisters and balconies of heavy, dark wood which would inspire gloom even in someone of an excessively cheerful disposition. (Until recently it was owned by the Wellcome Foundation and they manufactured Calpol in the grounds, vast volumes of the pink, gloopy mixture in huge steel vats like something out of *Charlie and the Chocolate Factory*. Today it is a chintzy hotel with patterned carpets and stiff, quilted bedspreads; how Lady Annabel would have turned.)

Her first husband, by whom she had five children, was killed in the First World War. She fell in love with my grandfather, Hugh Dodds, a handsome diplomat, brilliant horseman and elegant fencer. He came from a line of Scottish Covenanters, sons of the manse, so her family regarded him as irredeemably middle-class. Despite its objections, the couple married in 1922 when the bride was forty-one. My father, born four years later, was her seventh child but fifth son, hence his name, Quentin. Soon after he was sacked from Eton and just before he was sent down from Cambridge, the family changed from Dodds to Crewe. The official explanation is that for Annabel to inherit what was left of the estates after her father died in 1945, she had to add the name Crewe to her husband's. None of them liked the idea of a double-barrelled name and Hugh was not attached to his, so they changed it completely. Doubtless snobbish considerations also played a not insignificant part in the decision but I am not complaining. My mother always said that had Pop remained Quentin Dodds she would have called me Dorelia. He said if I had had a twin sister he would have called us Gonorrhoea and Syphilis, names he considered unusually pretty. I know Candida is a form of vaginal thrush but still feel, whatever way you look at it, it is preferable to a hardcore sexually transmitted disease. So if not Dorelia Dodds, I might have been Gonorrhoea Dodds or Syphilis Dodds. In the circumstances I think I got off lightly. (Incidentally, soon after Donovan and I got married, Pop happened to be browsing through a medical dictionary. He found listed there another STD, if a rather more obscure one, called Donovan's Bodies, and laughed for the whole afternoon.)

My father was a naturally spirited character and never one to toe lines. When not much older than a toddler, with his cherubic face and blond curls, he would be brought down from his bedroom to entertain his parents' guests with invented stories and merry recitations. As a young boy, living on the French Riviera where his father was Consul-General, he went to the Consulate one afternoon to meet him for a game of golf. A thin, blind man with a stick was waiting there and my father went to sit near him. The man explained to him he needed to see the Consul but the secretary told him it was not possible. Although the man's eyes were matt, he looked desperate. My father had never seen such an expression of desperation. The man told him he was Jewish and German. 'German to a schoolboy meant an enemy,' Pop later wrote in his memoirs, 'but this man was not an enemy.' He described his flight from the Gestapo and capture. His torturers had made him stand in front of a searchlight to force him to talk and it had burned out his eyes. He needed to get to England. My father begged his father to see the man. That day they 'got to golf a little late for once', but his mission was accomplished.

Later, at Eton, Pop was able to walk though he was lame and could not play games. He himself was spared the attention of bullies, perhaps because he was too easy a target, but he found the anti-Semitism, the taunting of Jewish boys, 'a hideous sight – the beginning, though, of unlearning. Unlearning about Jews; unlearning about [another boy's] mother in her cherry-bedecked hat being common . . . unlearning that money is important.' I have often wondered what it was about his character that enabled him to step

away from the prevailing view and judge that these preju-
dices were wrong. Perhaps it was an awareness of his own
vulnerability and the fact he had been spared the torment;
more likely it was empathy combined with an enlightened
courage and defiance born of a quick wit, a keen inquisi-
tiveness and optimism about the world. Whatever it was, it
meant he did not last long in that environment. (Out of
bravado or boredom he took off to London for the day and
was caught and 'encouraged' to leave.) During his sojourn at
the school he was beaten more than once for impertinence or
questioning rules that he thought were as unimaginative as
they were daft. It did not deter him. The skewering of
pomposity and highlighting the absurdity of bureaucracy
remained one of his favourite pastimes and, because he
always set about it with brilliance and humour, in later life
it extracted him from many a scrape with volatile officials in
hostile territories.

I have the impression he grew up with little sense of
belonging. This, alas, is something fiercely important to
me and at times my own failure to belong anywhere – in
a big family or amongst groups of friends – has caused me
pain. I wish I could have minded less especially as he came to
believe that it was not important and turned it to his
advantage, almost embraced it. I should have learned from
him. Certainly, from a young age I respected, almost hero-
worshipped him for his low opinion of it. As a child, I did not
know what it was exactly but I saw as something special his
difference from others, his aloofness from the crowd while at
the same time being very much a part of it, even its creator. It
was almost as if he was at the eye of a storm of his own
popularity and admiration but he existed according to his
own creed (though not a religious one – he was not a

churchgoer). His ability to turn his back from it and move away was something to which to aspire. Seen in a negative way, so wantonly not belonging could at times have been interpreted as a dodging of responsibility, such as the occasion when he took off in 1967 (I was three) for several months to cross the Empty Quarter (one of the very first Europeans ever to do so). I do not see it like that. It was bred, more, from an inspirational zest for life, a spirit of independence and adventure, a wish to experience the unknown, to learn about other cultures and befriend people so very different from himself. That is not to say he rejected his background. He was rebellious by nature but not a revolutionary. He enjoyed his membership of the establishment and was unexpectedly, in a few areas at least, a shocker of a snob. There were endless words I was never allowed to use. Toilet and pardon were just the beginning. Moist and settee featured on the extensive list which seemed to include many a word related to food – sweet (for pudding); dessert; cruet; condiment; cutlery; serviette; portion; sufficient, to name a few. It was the list with which he had been brought up, which bore a close resemblance to Nancy Mitford's, and which, though he is dead, I find I still cannot quite bring myself to use to this day lest I employ a tone that suggests I am doing so ironically. I know it is absurd.

But words were not the only thing which exercised his snobbery. He was proud of the fact his accent, while educated, was never preposterously plummy, but despite himself found he was unusually riled when my little half-brother and -sister (by his third wife) caught broad Staffordshire accents from primary school. And though his friends were from every background, he could often be heard decrying the 'ghastly' and 'pretentious' refinements of the middle classes as if he had forgotten, if his mother's family were to be taken seriously, that he was partly, 'irredeemably', middle-class himself.

As a young man, he virtually lived with Harold Macmillan and wholeheartedly fell in love with his daughter, Sarah, who later killed herself and whom, though he loved others deeply, he never quite forgot. Her mother, Lady Dorothy, used to gossip with him while sitting on the edge of his bath. His own mother died in 1953 when he was twenty-seven. Lady Violet Bonham-Carter has been described as a surrogate mother to him; her son, Mark, was my godfather. The way Pop saw it, his association with the aristocracy was part of him but not all. It did not preclude a relish of all that was new and imaginative – in terms of people from different backgrounds, of unpredictable political opinion, of innovative arts and ideas.

In the Sixties he was commissioned to go to South Africa to write an article about 'how things were getting better for the blacks and coloureds' but instead he reported how things under apartheid were getting so much worse. (He liked the fact that he was banned from re-entering the country for so many years.) Long before the vocabulary and practice of racism became unacceptable, he was with quiet dedication championing the cause against it. (Again, rather unexpectedly, there was an exception. He was rude about the Welsh. He must have felt they were alone in being fair game because I occasionally heard him speak about them in a derogatory way he never used about a single other nation.) When I was taught the song, 'Eeny, Meanie, Miney, Mo, Catch a Nigger by his Toe', in the school playground, without labouring the point he gently told me to replace the word 'nigger' with 'pobble'. He explained that a pobble was a mythical creature with no toes, so to say 'pobble' instead of 'nigger' would be to inject an element of wit into an otherwise tedious rhyme. When he was dying, two handsome young men – he always managed to land agreeable attendants who were patient beyond their years and full of adoration – were looking after him. One was South African, the other Irish. They left him a little too long in the bath. He dozed off and awoke rather cold. 'Oi, come here, you fucking revolutionaries,' he shouted at them, but after his own fashion, and in such a way that they just laughed and gave him a high five.

I knew there was something about him that was different from other fathers, and it was not just his wheelchair. (He had reluctantly succumbed to one in 1962. As he walked down the aisle with my mother, the congregation held its breath. He made it, just, with his walking-stick and without stumbling, but falling over was a regular occurrence in those days and he took the wheelchair on their honeymoon to Greece. I never saw him walking.)

For a start, he looked different. His sartorial sense was singular. Sombre pinstripes were not for him. One suit was brown with gold threads and, according to my mother, made him look like a comedian at the Palladium. He had some shirts with zips instead of buttons and wore kipper ties in acid-trip colours. (One was once displayed at the V&A as part of an exhibition in the Seventies: 'Fashion: An Anthology, by Cecil Beaton'.) At supper at home, kaftans from the Empty Quarter were his favoured choice, or his beloved embroidered dressing gown with a peach silk lining which he bought when he and his first wife, Martha, lived in Japan. He smoked cigarettes in long black or amber holders and we used to de-sludge them together with pipe cleaners as white as rabbits' tails. The molasses gunk that emerged was always startling. I was proud of him in every respect: his difference, his chair, his ties, even those cigarettes. At school one day we had to fill in a chart with the number of cigarettes our parents smoked. At five I delighted in putting sixty. It stood out. I was proud of his indomitable charm and a charisma which seemed to emanate from the fixed point of his wheelchair and sweep like dry ice across a room to touch people even in the furthest corners. At parties people would literally queue up to talk to him. He was a consummate raconteur and would tell the same anecdote a hundred times to different audiences and each telling would sound like a fresh telling. My half-brother and half-sister – whose mother was Martha – and I would roll our eyes and give each other looks as, in the latest company, we had to sit through the same story for the umpteenth time. But he always defied our scepticism and managed to make us laugh anew.

His own laugh, constrained somewhat by the weak muscles in his chest (muscular dystrophy causes the muscles throughout the body to crumble), was soft in sound but not in spirit. The lack of volume was made up for by shoulders that heaved and sometimes even tears that rolled down the cheeks. Employing the laborious movements of a seal on sand, straining a little and still heaving, he would quickly try to catch and dab the tears with his spotted linen handkerchief. I only once saw him shed real, sad tears and that was at the end of *The Glenn Miller Story*, when it was shown on the telly.

As I say, a throbbing snob in some respects, my father used to tease my mother about her less grand background, not because he minded but because he thought she did. The focus of his teasing was her maternal grandmother whose beginnings were relatively modest. Born in Dublin, her ambition in life was to achieve rich husbands. She managed to score and see off two of these and her double widowhood left her with the peculiar status of being the only woman in the 1950s to have a personal account at the Bank of England. She was, apparently, a monstrous woman, snobbish, vulgar and cruel. Her daughter, my grandmother, married young to get away from her but the chosen husband turned out to be an alcoholic. Granny divorced him sharpish on account of their incompatability, before marrying my very handsome grandfather, a 1930s Oscar-winning actor and later film producer. My grandparents lived in a claustrophobic flat in Belgravia. Although they always laughed a lot together throughout their marriage, they were an odd couple whose domestic arrangements were somewhat unconventional. Granny, who had aquamarine eyes, a sharp wit, a penchant for parties and more than her fair share of lovers, disappeared from the scene for several years when my mother and her sister were very young. They were brought up by their beloved father and equally loved old nanny. Mum adored and was inspired by her charismatic father – it was he who encouraged her to write. When Granny eventually returned Mum was twelve and resentful. She always disliked Granny's obsession with and endless rude comments about people's physical appearance. She regarded her as frivolous and superficial in almost every way but not least in her opinion that educated women were bluestockings. Mum regrets to this day that Granny would not allow her to go to university and forced her instead to become an unwilling debutante.

After coming out, Mum started to earn her living as a journalist. She met my father, who was thirteen years older than her, whilst working as a lowly caption-writer on *Queen* magazine. He was there in a rather loftier position. They married and after two years in a ground-floor flat in west London they moved to the William and Mary house in Wootton with which they fell in love but could not for the life of them afford. They must have been madly optimistic or just plain mad. It was never going to last long.

He was a freelance writer. My mother, who was in her early twenties, was working flat-out to help pay the bills. She was a reporter at BBC television on a documentary series called *Man Alive*. She reluctantly commuted to London daily in her lilac Triumph. I used to stand on the kitchen window-sill howling for her as I saw her car turn out of the drive, breath and distress besmirching the gelid glass. She was beautiful. Whenever I have asked anyone about their child-hoods I have been impressed that, without exception, all have said their mothers were beautiful. Perhaps all mothers just are and mine was no exception. To me she was supremely loving and gaspingly beautiful. I was not aware of a warmer or more glamorous woman alive. Her presence, her affection and that warmth, was what I lived for. Her glamour dazzled as far as the wan horizon of industrial chimneys. She wore silk headscarves which she tied in a loose knot beneath her chin and which made her face look thin. She had miniskirts, wide belts with outsize tortoise-shell clasps and an eighteen-inch waist to maintain. She was famous in her circle for that waist. Even her knuckles were sleek. They had sophisticated bones inside them whereas, when I flattened my hands, all mine had were demeaning dimples. And in her cupboard there were black suede shoes with what I took for real diamond buckles. When she had gone to London, I used to sneak upstairs and open that cupboard. I would cautiously shake the thin polythene shrouds protecting her soft, bright clothes so as to smell the smell of her stephanotis toilet water as it jolted free. I most vividly remember the cream, thick-corduroy minidress; a crotch-length pink cotton gingham one; a black silk jersey number, heavy, with silk jersey buttons running all the way down the back like an orderly queue of beetles. And I would touch the supposed diamonds on those shoes – they glittered even in the recesses of the cupboard's dark interior till I was brought back downstairs again and fed a consoling biscuit.

My father had happened by chance upon the job of a restaurant critic and became rather serious about food. Being in a wheelchair he needed someone to help him, and he employed a man called Chris whose wife, Edgy, was an excellent cook with a particular talent for quiche lorraine (never was there a creamier version than Edgy's in all the world) and ginger cake dark and dank as boot polish. Her absolute speciality, though, was very precocious for its day – a hedgehog pudding of poached meringue with roasted almond spines and a sauce called crème anglaise. She had a Pekinese called Fellah and once gave me a round of Roger & Gallet's carnation soap, not much larger than a coin, which I never opened because I liked too much the tiny box and label with its little picture of the flowers, red and pink. One birthday, her card to me had on the front an illustration of kittens making merry at a tea party, with tiny sausages, chocolate biscuits and jellies laid out on their table. The cup cakes had that same carnation combination of red and pink, pink icing with red cherries on top. The smell of that soap and any sight of those colours together transports me back to Edgy's cooking – our kitchen with its groovy tiles, shiny white formica, and chunky Kenwood mixer – and my earliest memories of food.

*   *   *

I would say that my relationship with food as a child differed little from that of any other child's. I had things I loved: fish pie, cottage pie, roast chicken, apple crumble, Sainsbury's cream cheese on plain digestives and – no surprises here – cakes and sweets and biscuits too. I had things I loathed – no surprises here either: parsnips, spinach and leeks and almost every type of cheese. I wasn't allowed to eat what I loved most all the time, and wasn't always made to eat what I loathed. My parents, liberal Sixties types who had no wish to impose their more draconian kinds of upbringings on me, were not unreasonable. It was never, you'll sit there till you've finished your cold frog-spawn tapioca, even if it means you're there till tea. There was only one negative incident with food – we all have one, don't we, encrusted on the mind? – that I suppose came close. It was of being sent by my mother to the end of a cold corridor with a plate of leeks and strict instructions not to return till they were all gone. I did not have the wit to bend out of the back door and scrape them down a willing drain. Instead I stood with that damn plate, my whole being heaving and retching at each laborious mouthful into a long and gruesome afternoon. By rights, I should not be able to abide the very sight of a leek to this day, but as it happens I can eat them; I bear no such grudge.

I often ate what my parents ate, and what they always ate was very good food that, because of my father's occupation, tended to be fresh, imaginative, cosmopolitan, ahead of its time. My mother's paperback copies of Elizabeth David's books were yellowing, curling, thumb-greased and stained with Venn-diagram rings from the burgundy bottoms of wine glasses past. I was spoilt. If it wasn't spaghetti, it was spaghetti soufflé, for God's sake. And this in the days when a large proportion of the population of all England could believe, as became evident so famously one April Fool's Day, that spaghetti grew on trees. No wonder I enjoyed eating and had a tummy distended by more than my liver. My mother and father used to tease me about my stomach. Quite often they would lift my T-shirt or dress and snuffle their faces into my warm round flesh to make me laugh. And laugh I did, with the genuine joy of knowing they loved it and me. There again, my father had two adjectives which, now and then when he was testy, he used to call me – lazy and greedy. Individually they cut deep, much more so than disobedient, cheeky or stubborn ever could. But together they were even worse because, together, they joined in an unholy matrimony of objectionable fat.

My parents had a huge bathroom with a vista of carpet, walk-in cupboards, an armchair and bidet and tall, wide windows overlooking the lawn. It could have been a drawing room. I spent many an hour in there. My father's morning routine was a long one. It was coffee and toast and marmalade amongst the linen sheets of his bed, followed by a leisurely bath during which he liked to have company. I used to sit in his wheelchair beside the bath, talking to him as he lay there washing his face with a soapy flannel and sinking down deep to rinse his hair. We talked about all sorts of things and he would top up the water by turning the old-fashioned hot tap with his toes. Getting out of the bath was something of a business so we used to put it off as long as possible. He told me funny stories and gossiped cheerfully. When he finally consented to being hauled out by my mother, I helped to dry him and get him dressed. I would watch as he cleaned his teeth with an electric toothbrush he seemed somehow to have obtained before they were invented and 'flossed' his teeth with a strange water-squirting system involving a cream plastic box and a small hose. I brushed his hair back with an ivory-handled brush engraved with his initials and only then were we ready to enter the lift.

We used to go down together in the lift between the bathroom and the library on the ground floor where he worked. It was a noisy, cumbersome old thing which had been specially installed for him and into which he and his wheelchair and I only just fitted if I pressed myself tightly against its dark wooden side. He let me snap the dull gold grille shut and press the green plastic button – never the red one – and the whole creaky contraption would groan into life and start to wheeze and judder downwards in a stately manner towards the square of concrete at the bottom of the shaft. The lift's underside was a flat, grey surface made of what looked like thick suede. It had clods of dust round the edges and was filled with air and wobbled as the lift made its uneasy progress either up or down. It acted as a kind of sensor which meant that when it touched the ground the lift automatically stopped. In fact if it touched anything, however insignificant and even something neither firm nor flat, the lift would, for safety reasons, immediately come to a halt.

One morning after bath-time, I must have been about four, my father suggested I should go downstairs ahead of him and stand in the lift shaft to try it out. When the lift's sensitive bum landed on my head the whole thing would grind to a halt, or at least it should if it was as safe as Otis claimed it was. I thought it was a brilliant idea and enthusiastically did as he said. I ran down, went to the corner of the library and stepped on to the patch of concrete at the bottom of the shaft.

'Ready?' my father bellowed from directly above me.

'Ready!'

'Coming!'

I heard the familiar grill and groan of the lift's lift-off and looked upwards to see its wobbling square bottom steadily making its way towards my head. I watched loops of cable slithering like dreary snakes at the back wall of the shaft and shivered with the delight of our thrilling experiment. As the couple of tons of lift, wheelchair and father inched closer I hunched my shoulders and couldn't look any more. I squeezed my eyes tight with irresistible fear. I could detect the weight nudging closer, same as you can sense a person looking at you even if you cannot see them. Then I felt a faint pat on the crown of my head and heard the sound of the mechanism's sharp halt. It had worked! Triumphantly I bent out from underneath the lift which had been arrested three or four feet or so (whatever my height was at the time) from its landing pad, and my father and I congratulated ourselves on our feat and laughed and laughed.

It became our party trick. Whenever there were guests to stay we would make them assemble in the library when Pop was ready to come down. I would take up my position in the lift shaft and they would be made to watch as my father descended and for all the world was about to crush the living daylights out of me.

My mother was rather less keen but, boy, did my father and I love that trick. We used to do it often and relish the appalled reactions and horrified shrieks of all the onlookers until one day, when I was not in the shaft, the mechanism carried on even when the lift and my father in it touched the ground. Although my father arranged for the lift to be mended, from then onwards he deemed our game too risky for us to continue playing it. I was distraught.

'But what if you were underneath and it didn't stop one day?' he reasoned. 'You'd be squished flat as a pancake.'

We did not do it again.

My half-brother and -sister, respectively six and five years older than me, lived with their mother in London and I did not see them often. I was alone but I was not lonely. Though my parents were working hard there were plenty of other adults around for company. I sat on the lap of silver-haired Doris in the dining room to help her polish the silver and she rewarded me with old-lady hugs that smelt of her Yardley-powdery skin, her Bronnley soap and her laundry. Edgy let me stir the Christmas pudding in a vast basin till my arms ached and the dark fruit and sixpences made sucking noises with the sloshes of brandy. I always had nannies and liked them. I remember Sylvia, who smoked like one of the chimneys at the nearby brickworks, and, after her, Australian Maureen, whose sharp fingernails dug into my skin as she washed my face and who once pinned a note on my back saying, 'Beware, I bite.' They used to drive me to local dance classes in a sickly green Morris Minor. The car, with its comforting smell emanating from the cracks in the matching leather seats, its lively indicator stick which flashed orange at the end and metal glove compartment with its sharp handle that looked like a mouth, seemed to have a character all of its own and, until the crash which scarred my eye, felt like something I could befriend.

There was also my governess. To this day I find it remarkable that such a thing still existed in my lifetime and that I had one. That was how my parents referred to her but she was really just a retired teacher who, when I was too young to go to school, came in a few mornings a week to teach me to read and write at a wooden school desk in the nursery. I liked Mrs Robinson. She was a kindly woman with a bag of star stickers in all the colours of the rainbow, including mauve. (I remember them well because I did not score many and those I did were much-prized.) And there was Becky. I went to Becky's modern house in the village to play with our dolls. My mother has a serious doll phobia, bad as other people have for snakes or spiders, so my Sindy was not allowed to put in much of an appearance at home, however elegantly I dressed her in green needle-cord smocks. To give her full rein I had to take her to my friend's house, till my friend, same age as me, nearly died of pneumonia and had to stay for a long time in hospital where I was not allowed to visit her. Or I occasionally visited Ron and Amy, an elderly couple who did odd jobs for my parents. In his garage, Ron often used to respray my father's ludicrous purple car because it landed more than its fair share of bumps and scrapes. As I swung on the old yellow swing in their garden listening to the rusty scratch of its handles, I could smell the rich smell of that spray and wanted to drink it. Inside, Ron and Amy's front room had a gas fire and three-piece suite next to which stood, on a stirring carpet, a thin, plywood, two-dimensional figure of a man. He was black, painted to look a bit like one of the golliwogs which appeared for too many years on jars of jam. He had a fetching smile and wore a butler's suit, with stripy trousers and shiny shoes. He was leaning forward slightly, a real metal ashtray in his upturned hands and, much the same size as me, he became my friend. I think I called him Pip. I used to have long conversations with him. Then I would hear the flap of the coloured plastic ribbons which hung for reasons I could not fathom from the top of the door through to the kitchen and which I longed to have in our house but instinctively knew my mother would not go for. The flapping would hail the appearance of Amy, who would step through them to bring me back, feet tapping on patterned lino, to the fug by the range for high tea of cottage pie and home-made jam tarts.

I learned early to invent characters in my head or out of incidental figures like Pip or anything else available to me. One day I pulled petals off several roses in the garden and built a house for them on the grass out of old bricks. I was given a toy shop with a wooden façade and would stand behind its counter for hours, writing lists on its blackboard, talking to imaginary customers and ringing up their plastic coins in the till. The groceries, just a few inches high, were replicas of real ones. There were red, yellow and blue tins of Bird's Custard which I had never eaten or even come across in real life but which nevertheless seemed to convey to me a homely feel. There were minuscule packets of cornflakes, tubs of hot chocolate and boxes of jelly and Atora, along with a whole variety of other familiar brands in all their diminutive glory. I hadn't a clue what Atora was – still haven't; suet? – but its box had pleasing stripes. In fact my whole stock was more than pleasing; it was irresistible. I could pass entire mornings piling every item neatly on the wooden shelves and bossing my make-believe customers about, telling them which ones they should and shouldn't buy. It was my favourite game and only ever gave way to the odd television programme such as *Play School*, *Hector's House*, *Camberwick Green* or *Watch with Mother* – which I really did watch with mine. We would nestle together on the funky nursery sofa which was red with pink psychedelic flowers that looked like those sticking out of Ermintrude's mouth in *The Magic Roundabout*. I smelt her stephanotis and felt the warmth of her beside me and could not have asked for more.

I started at nursery school and made friends there, I suppose, though all I actually remember about it is an episode with chocolate biscuits. It was on the long drive home following my performance in the nativity play. I had played the part of the angel's mother, or so I told my own mother, and she had been so proud of me that she overlooked the fact that I had got away with one too many milk chocolate digestives. Although I was in the front seat I was massively car sick all over my navy woollen tights. A couple of decades later I went on officially to become a bulimic, but that was one of the first and last times in my life that I ever threw up.

I was still about four, sitting with my mother as she sorted through the linen cupboard at the top of the wide wooden stairs. She had inherited lots of old sheets, waxy in their softness, from her spinster aunt, some with embroidered initials, JS, for Jenny Simpson. There were others too, newer than Aunt Jenny's, with my parents' initials, A and Q, in my mother's beloved lilac, and a large C joining them, masquerading as an ampersand. There was also a whole set of lilac towels, similarly initialled. Wedding presents. As my mother kneeled in one of her miniskirts before the piles and took them out to tidy and order them, she told me she would give them to me when I got married. Another day, at her clothes cupboard, her hands passed over her wedding dress, a duchesse satin one she had designed herself, with a rib-tight bodice; tiny. I could have this for my wedding day, she said, if I liked. And her eighteen-inch waist, could I have that too?

*   *   *

45

In 1969, I was five, my mother and father divorced. I wondered about those sheets and towels, their fate. But I did know that as long as they existed my parents would always retain a link, if only one embroidered on to a set of bath towels.

They divorced, my father later wrote in his autobiography, 'in sorrow, certainly not in anger'; Mum had been targeted 'by someone of no importance', a volatile character who had a hold over her based wholly on her fear of his bullying. A few weeks later, according to my father, she telephoned him early one morning.

'She was in Brighton,' Pop wrote. 'She said she was about to get married, in ten minutes. I pleaded with her. She cried and rang off.' (The photographs show her looking fantastic in a black, wild, wet-look minicoat with thigh-high boots to match and huge, very dark, dark glasses.) 'That afternoon,' my father continued, 'she came to my flat in London. She said she had done it. She couldn't help it. I said that she could get an annulment and I would remarry her. It was impossible.'

Myself, I remember nothing of the divorce or any of this. Perhaps I have blocked out the memories because they are too painful. Certainly that would fit with the modern obsession of reading psychological trauma into every negative experience suffered by every individual. It does not fit, though, with what is much more likely, in my case at any rate, to be the – rather more mundane – truth. As it happens, I do not think I found the divorce painful, certainly not enough to have merited blocking it out. I remember nothing of it because I was supremely fortunate in as much as my parents were able conscientiously to protect me from their distress and remained full of respect for each other. They never once refused to speak. Quite the opposite. They spoke often, always fondly, and without bitterness or vengeance, and, I like to suppose, only with regret. As a result I was able to accept the new status quo without questioning it, so there is nothing much to remember. Adults often credit children with extraordinary resilience in the face of searing events and rightly so in many cases. But I do not think I was remotely resilient. That did not come into it. I went along with the new arrangements just in the way children do, thinking they were normal, or not really thinking about them at all.

Our house at Wootton was sold. I literally kissed it goodbye. Mum was crying and crying as we left and has since told me I was much braver than her. I wasn't. I just did not fully understand. We moved to London. She lived for a while in a friend's studio flat in Chelsea which had a vast white furry rug and a round kitchen table with one central leg, the whole thing made of white moulded plastic. I visited her there and we went on happy outings to a brilliant, innovative shop called Kids in Gear where, on different occasions, she bought me a lilac T-shirt with an open neck and creamy buttons, lime-green jeans, red shiny clogs with silver studs, a purple satin shirt with outsize collar and luminous sleeves, jerseys with striped sleeves in rainbow colours and a rich-red velvet waistcoat covered on the front with a mosaic of mirrors, each one the size of a halfpenny. Or maybe Kids in Gear came later. Either way, I did not live with Mum but we had great times on our own together – shopping (I enjoyed it in those days), going to the cinema (*Fantasia* was the first film I ever saw, and *The Red Balloon* at the ICA), eating at hamburger joints like the Great American Disaster (corn and cucumber relishes, on a miniature carousel, a tremendous novelty) – times that were as precious as any I can remember.

There were no custody battles or lawyers. I lived with my father for several months because, under the new circumstances, it was considered by him and Mum to be a better option. But it cannot have been very convenient for him and must have been more than vexing for his new wife, my stepmother Sue, to have a spoilt five-year-old and a nanny in her midst. Sue was just twenty and full of humour, exuberance and vitality. Sometimes her hair was purple, sometimes green. She wore platforms and velvet kaftans in rich colours with beautiful dull-gold embroidery. They had married in a Register Office. A guest at the reception convinced me he could turn me into a frog. I knew that in France they ate frogs' legs, my father had told me so, and was faintly alarmed; otherwise I forget the occasion, except for Sue and her numerous lively siblings who were kind to me, funny and warm.

My father and Sue, the nanny and I all lived in Kensington in a dark, ground-floor flat – bought with my father's wheelchair in mind – in a Fifties block with cold, metal window frames. The kitchen at the back, overlooking a dreary communal courtyard, was darkened by a huge, rusty fire escape just outside its window. The bathroom, its brown wallpaper patterned with shiny gold shapes, had no window at all and was darker still. Every evening I played 'Beggar my Neighbour' with my father for half an hour or so before he and Sue went out. Sometimes he tried to teach me to tie a bow or tell the time and frightened me with his impatience if – as was invariably the case – I failed to grasp the concepts. Left and right was a particular heel. 'Oh, so *stupid*,' he would say when, rabbit in the headlights, I would get them wrong for the umpteenth time. 'You know the difference between up and down, for God's sake, why not left and right?' More often I sat on his lap and he read to me, *The Wind in the*

48

Willows, and that was joyous. During the day, when he was writing and I was home from school, I spent many an hour in my room playing 'Heart of Gold' or 'Bridge Over Troubled Water' again and again and again on a box gramophone with a grey plastic lid. I found using the tiny lever to lift the little arm and return the needle to the beginning of the record an extremely satisfying pastime, even if, despite so much repetition, the actual words of the songs left me hopelessly bemused. I realise, looking back through my interpretation of Simon and Garfunkel's *Cecilia*, that though my parents may have been married three times each and the tribulations of their lives occasionally given me pause, I led a shamefully sheltered life. I thought, 'Oh, Cecilia you're breaking my heart, you're shaking my confidence daily,' referred to someone shaking a cleaner, a bit like Tony sometimes shook me and my Mum. But unlike me, this mythical daily, who in my mind's eye looked like silver-haired Doris, had the advantage of confidence and for that I rather envied her.

I adored my new school; the last one I ever did.

I was lucky to get into it. When my mother went to meet the headmistress to see if there was a last-minute place for me due to our change of circumstance, I was made to wait for a while in a classroom of girls and boys my age. They were being taught English and I was transfixed. Mum reappeared with Mrs Garnsey after twenty minutes or so and I jumped up. 'Can I come to this school?' I asked. They shook their heads. There were no spaces.

'Great. That's no home, no father, and now no school,' I apparently replied with precocious melodrama, and on over-hearing this Mrs Garnsey said to Mum, 'The child can start on Monday.'

The school was a rabbit warren behind the elegant façade of two or three large stucco houses haphazardly knocked together on Holland Park Avenue. The classrooms were cramped, linked by small creaking stairs and narrow corridors along which were tracks of pegs bulging with duffel coats, gym bags and striped woollen scarves. Everywhere there was a smell of damp and feet and catering steam which oozed into the felt uniform and which we daily took home with us as surely as our satchels. The two tarmac playgrounds at the back were tiny. But we did not notice. An undeveloped sense of scale made them seem perfectly big to me.

I liked the teachers, who were young and warm. I went on tea dates with girls and played with their dolls, tea dates with boys and looked at blood on glass slides under the simplistic metal microscopes they had been given for Christmas. I embraced the poetry and drama, even the recorder which came in a beige corduroy pouch and the screeches of which could never become music. The place was homely, comforting, fun, and I used to run along the pavement each morning to its wrought iron gate and duck down the stone steps into the peeling basement cloakroom.

The school had just one fault. The food. Dark Age discs of beetroot with geological ridges. Thinner discs of smooth Spam, texture of a damp swab and the startling colour of baby lotion on the outside, with a compacted circle of etiolated stuffing – if that's what it was? – within. Jaundiced salad cream that pulled off the feat of being both sharp and sickly at the same time. Pale pink custard, its congealed skin, when picked off with a fork, like the soft, viral bullet from a sneeze. It was completely unmanageable. I could not eat it and did not. Like many resourceful children down the ages, confronted with similar fare, when the teacher wasn't looking I shoved it up my skirt, down my knickers and afterwards into the jaws of an appreciative lavatory. It wasn't rocket science but I remember the sense of achievement at having managed to do it without detection, as well as a sense of virtue, less explicable, about not having eaten at all. I can't think I felt virtuous then for the same reasons I do today when I skip a meal. I was five. But it must have been related to the notion that calorific denial is somehow good. The hollow feeling, mid-afternoon, even then was gently compelling. And, once I got home, which was now with my mother, I was definitely aware of the added pleasure and regret of endless eggy bread that Mum and I would toast in a frying pan of butter for our tea without Tony. My new stepfather – a film director who had met Mum at the BBC – was thankfully always too preoccupied to join in, pacing the kitchen, scooting his blunt finger for dust along high-up surfaces, and shouting.

After nine months or so with my father and Sue at Cottesmore Court, I had moved to live with Mum and Tony. I don't know why the change but I was so happy to be with her again. I had missed her with a vacuum in the stomach which felt a whole heap more intense than the hollowness of merely missing lunch. She had bought for peanuts – it was 1969 and the area was still a long way from being preposterous – a large, derelict flat on the top floor of a house in Holland Park and done it up with her usual flair, colourfully and cosily. She had mauve wallpaper in her and Tony's bedroom and in the sitting room a huge, bright yellow rug with white splodges and fat knots from a fashionable Spanish shop in Pimlico called Casa Pupo. There was a smaller version, same style only purple, in the bathroom. After a few months we moved up the road to a socking great house in a square with a communal garden, and my stepfather played music so loud the whole place shook and my mother went deaf in one ear. It was in the white formica kitchen in that house that Mum and I ate our eggy bread and she patiently tested me on my spellings, to the ever-present thuds and slams of the Rolling Stones coming from Tony's skyscraper hi-fi in the drawing room above or his cutting room in the basement.

Sometimes my father took me to lunch at new restaurants. Many were Italian with pink linen tablecloths, hard bread rolls and crinkly packets of grissini. A favourite of his was in the Fulham Road and called San Frediano. The ebullient chef, his stomach the size of a small Mediterranean island, always used to appear in his whites to greet us. Children weren't very welcome in restaurants in those unenlightened days, but the Italian in him – or the knowledge of which side his ciabatta was oiled – would always welcome me. He once presented me with an orchid and showed me round his kitchens. Whenever I went there or anywhere else with my father, I always ordered the same food. Prawn cocktail and *pollo surpriso*. I could never tire of cutting into the cheeky, breaded breast of chicken for that maternal outpouring of melted butter with parsley flecks, of watching it pooling on to the oval white plate. Sitting in the crisp, grown-up environment of those Seventies restaurants, alone with my father, being treated like an adult, there was nothing for it but to be happy.

It was the same at Netherset, the Staffordshire dairy farm near Crewe that my father and Sue moved to, as it had been at Wootton. Like my mother, Sue had never boiled an egg before getting married but shortly afterwards was making Peking duck (deliriously exotic for Stoke-on-Trent circa 1970), damson cheese and, to go with raspberries, a startling sweet cream infused with geranium leaves that tasted gloriously of greenhouses.

Aged five and onwards, I ate all this wondrous food and continued to contribute to my solidly laid foundations not of huge fatness but of a definite softness round the edges. Alas, I was not the outdoor type who enjoyed burning it all off. Going on walks to nowhere in the cold and the wind (at which Staffordshire excelled) always seemed to me an activity of supreme discomfort and pointlessness. When my father suggested I went for a walk, I felt he did so in the spirit of wanting to get me out of the house. I'm sure he thought I would enjoy it too, but I don't think I was entirely wrong about his need to get rid of me. He had to work, after all. Walks, solitary or otherwise, took on the wintry hue of banishment, if not exactly punishment, as opposed to pleasure.

It was not only the nagging notion that I was unwanted. It was not the physical trial of walking, one step in front of another, which I minded, but *a* walk. If a walk was a piece of clothing, it would be a hair shirt. There is apparently virtue to be derived from going on one. Walks are good for you, as my father so often used to remind me. That quasi-biblical combination of fresh air, exercise, nature. But they never felt good to me. Invariably, a walk meant a bleak landscape, spooky black branches, mud sucking and gluing, cows with expressionless eyes and dismissive tails, even the odd pissed-off bull or, on the downs above my mother's cottage in Wiltshire, a dead sheep in a stone trough of water from which I was about to drink. It meant hair whipping my face (even if tied up, it always broke loose), running eyes and streaming red nose, thick layers that did nothing to protect me from the cold and yet were bulky and achy to move inside; a cold sweat, then discarded jumpers so tedious to carry. With companions, it meant being humiliatingly silenced by a steep hill due to lack of breath; on one's own, amidst all that hostile nature, it meant a loneliness fit to burst.

I absolutely hated walks, and don't relish the prospect of going on one to this day, except that I am now of an age to appreciate nature more, the sweep and detail of seasons. If I go on a walk today it is not to make me feel better. What is this better? Depends how you define it.

But it's not just walks. No form of exercise has ever held any appeal for me. I don't know why my body is so unresponsive to physical exertion. The act of swimming, running, playing tennis or working out in the gym never gives me that elusive high which sporting types so exhort, and has never done all the things to me that others swear by. I once talked to an objectionable physical training instructor in the RAF. He had little time for civilians and even less for ones like me who enjoy sitting by the fire with newspapers and cups of hot chocolate. He nastily referred to our ilk as Fat Jobbers. I am a Fat Jobber par excellence. I really hate gyms. Like Colman's is said to make the big money not out of the mustard that people eat but from that which they leave in a blob on their plates, so gyms cynically make their money from blobs like me who join in the spirit of optimism and quickly lapse in the slough of despond. Not wanting to part with any money that would sure as eggs is eggs be wasted, in early 1992, as a New Year's resolution, I took up running. People told me it would make me feel more energetic, less tired, and would increase my mental alertness. They said it would only take two weeks for me to begin to feel the benefits. I was sceptical but started anyway because I wanted to lose weight. I believe most women's main motivation, though they may kid themselves otherwise, for going in for such an unreasonable activity must be their weight.

For five months I ran five days a week and every run had me retching for breath. Yet I carried on doggedly because therein, I thought, weight loss lay. I persisted for another seven months, determined to shift those pounds. The running became a little easier, sometimes, and the bath at the end of it was always good. But what I felt as it became marginally less painful was vague curiosity, never pleasure. In all that time, a whole year, on just two occasions was I even aware I was fit. Once, skiing, I found I could walk up a mountain jauntily, skis slung over my shoulder, and that I own was useful. On another occasion, walking up a hill in Provence with two girlfriends, I did not become out of breath for a moment, and that felt good. I didn't lose weight, but guess I didn't put on as much as I might have done had I not been running. I never once felt 'better'. I felt exactly the same.

I decided to cut the labour of the run and go directly to the bath. Strictly, I don't need the Radox or equivalent muscle relaxant any more but I allow myself the luxury of a few bubbles and the bath is still good. Nowadays, if I can help it, I never run, barely go on walks at all and certainly never move in the sustained sort of way which requires special shoes.

'And as anyone could have foretold, her marriage soon ended,' my father wrote of Mum's misguided second union. In 1972, I was seven, she made her excuses, as they say, and left him. It was to a cottage in Wiltshire that she and I at last escaped. She found it, a tuppenny wreck, and worked her magic upon it. He stalked her awhile but was soon diverted by another unfortunate target. Thereafter Mum and I were alone, safe together and relieved.

I look back at the period before Mum and I arrived at our cottage and try to find there the seeds of my fragile relationship with weight and food. I can find none, or none that are completely plausible. At Wootton, Cottesmore Court and Netherset, yes, my father used to tell me every so often that I was greedy. I accept that these remarks hurt and contributed to a certain sensitivity about greed and its consequences, but cannot help wondering if as an explanation for lifelong food worries it is not rather simplistic and feeble. They were a contributing factor, merely. I feel the same about my parents' divorce and new marriages and the ripple effects of moving house and school. I suppose they must have been a contributing factor too but I remain puzzled as to how exactly. I missed Mum and felt that missing as a continual dead weight in my stomach, but I do not have any recollection of being grossly upset or traumatised. There is a black and white photograph of me at the time, taken by her. I am wearing a Kids in Gear T-shirt and staring out of the window of her rented studio flat. The expression on my face is searingly sad; I look like my entire family has just been executed, but I am not convinced. I had probably just mislaid a toy a few moments before or finished a tube of Smarties; at worst I had just been told it was time to leave her and go back to Cottesmore Court. I could not say with any certainty that that expression revealed deep sadness at my situation. That would be too pat and unreliable an interpretation. I was actually very lucky in as much as Pop and Mum remained on excellent terms, continued happily to talk to and see each other, and when I was still living with him I never went for very long without seeing her.

I was never aware of rows and atmospheres and, even if I had been, who is to say the tensions and fears arising from those would have been translated into a deep dislike of my belly, hips and thighs? The divorce was unusually civilised and to me at the time felt like an adventure, rather exciting, not troubling, not grounds for guilt and self-hatred. When I reached an age at which I fully understood and might have been upset about it, the new set-up was already part of the fabric of my life. By then a so-called conventional or nuclear family life, without step-parents and half-siblings I loved, would have been hard to imagine. I suppose in an ideal world I should have liked my mother and father to have remained married, for them to have gone on living and having more children together, but I never saw much point in lingering overly long on the hypothetical. As it was their complicated arrangements added colour, or so it seemed to me, and made for a family more varied and extended than most. Whenever I met people they were always very intrigued and asked me to explain how it worked. Their curiosity made me feel pleased, flattered almost. It gave me a sense of not being ordinary. It was not a straightforward family but I could not think of it as a bad thing.

Mrs McCombie sat at the head of the large, battered table in her stifling kitchen and never moved. Her industrial range gave rise to the perennial outburst of sweat across her brow, upon which the overhead neon strip bestowed a sickly shine. Laid out in front of her were two plastic crates. One had little milk bottles and silver tops, the other long white buns topped with icing that was Persil white or Andrex pink. We queued to take one of each and enjoy her specialist subject of Scottish teasing. It was the routine every break-time for the three years I was at that school near Salisbury, and not a day passed without my staring at her phenomenal flesh and being taken aback yet again by its expanse. The flesh of her calves, with its patina of purple, buckled and folded over her ankles like fallen trousers so that only the toes of her put-upon slippers showed beneath. The blatant nylon of her patterned summer dresses stretched across the breathless landscape of her amorphous bosom and the push of her open knees. Her favoured style of dress, with its lack of sleeves, made for a revelation of dimpled upper arm with a circumference equal to that of a punchbag. I had never seen such fat. It was more than intriguing. It was riveting.

I stared then as I still stare now, though I hope more subtly, at people who are fat. This is an admission which sticks in my throat; more, it actually frightens me to voice it because I am so ashamed of it. People with facial disfigurements or withered limbs or squints or birthmarks or hunchbacks or unusual disabilities speak of being stared at, but not by me. I used to stroll along beside my father in his wheelchair and when passers-by stared at him his dignity breezily ignored them. I could not. I felt contempt for their base curiosity and vowed never to sink so low, but I'm no better. I've harboured my own base curiosity about fat people, equally contemptuous, long as I can remember. I cannot keep my eyes off them. There is no digression from the norm which fascinates me more than obesity. First, because it is a state which, nominally at any rate, has about it a level of choice, and second, because at certain – admittedly brief and irrational – moments in my life I have felt quite close to it myself. Times in my life when I have convinced myself that the stares I am engendering on the bus or at the checkout are due to my own mesmerising size. I didn't blame the starers. If I spot a really fat man or woman – but especially woman – in the street, I find myself watching them till they turn the corner or slip out of sight. I watch exactly how the fat is laid about them because fat is so imaginative and cunning and diverse in how it chooses to cover a body. The uniform of fat is interpreted differently by every individual who wears it. For some, the stomach is the main feature, or the hips and thighs; for others, the face and neck and upper arms and calves; for more still, the buttocks and back, the tops of feet, the backs of hands and wrists. Any combination, or all of the above, and every inch of fat shaped differently, its very folds and creases moving and falling in unique and mysterious ways.

I find myself looking, looking and speculating. I try to gauge the person's nationality, background, marital status and state of mind. I know my own preoccupation with fat. The people I stare at are fatter than me – so what must be their preoccupation? Every sleeping as well as waking moment? Was there some trauma that brought them to their current weight, or was it nothing simpler than an ebullient enjoyment of food? Or maybe they are not in the least preoccupied? I scrutinise the face for signs of distress or indifference. If they look miserable, I arrogantly assume it's because they are fat even though I have not the faintest idea and it's none of my business. If they are smiling, why, it's because they are putting on a brave face of course. From where I'm standing, someone can't be that fat *and* happy. The two don't go together. When I was at my fattest I could fake happy with every bit as much aplomb as Sally faked her orgasm in that restaurant with Harry. But genuine happy I could not muster. I also wonder about the choice of clothes, such vistas of stretchy material: where they were bought, whether the changing room on the day of purchase gave rise to any feelings of anxiety, panic or self-loathing, or if that is my own unforgivable projection? I think about what might be their favourite food, how they eat it – alone, and how much? How *much*? If they are eating an apple or sandwich when I see them, or more amazingly, a McDonald's or chocolate bar, I marvel at their courage. Even today, I don't really like eating on the street, let alone something famously seething with calories. I'm too cowardly. It's a leftover from what I used to think: that I couldn't brave the infinite eyes shouting, no wonder I'm fat, it's high time a greedy fat pig like me WENT ON A DIET. I think about the logistics of sex. Unwelcome pictures form in the mind which I desperately try to shake off. I ask myself about issues of navigation. How anything shorter than a horse's penis can make it round that stomach, between those thighs, and how come it does not lose its way?

I suppose I hadn't been too sorry to leave London and my primary school behind to transfer to the boarding school where Mrs McCombie was the cook. As a child I could not believe a person could be so big. Mrs McCombie was one human being and yet it seemed to me there was enough of her for three.

Boarding school specialised in midnight feasts, and beetroot and Spam, I knew, were not midnight-feast fare. Consolation, indeed, for moving from the city, my home, my lovely school and my friends. Midnight feasts and pillow fights beckoned. Before I went there I had never heard the word homesick.

I soon did. Within hours. And manifestly discovered the full force of its meaning. I had just turned eight. The lino on all the floors, colour of cow-pats, was cold and attracted dawn mists of dust beneath our beds. The horse hair in our mattresses mournfully moaned as we turned in the night. Bats circled the ceiling of our dormitory and threatened to lose themselves in our hair as a flapping knot of nightmares. To avoid them, and the inevitable sound and smell of someone in the next door bed being copiously homesick into a scratched enamel bowl, I used to head to the bottom of my bed with my fingers in my ears, repeating, 'rhubarb, rhubarb'. The teachers and matrons were kind and affectionate, for the most part. They smiled and joked and put their arms round us at the first sign of failure, triumph or tears but they were not our mothers. There was one telephone in the school, in the staff room, which our parents could ring only on our birthdays and in the event of family tragedy. Not being able to see my mother let alone talk to her felt to me much the same as it would have done had she been untimely ripped from this life by a car crash. The hollow ache of loss lingered in my stomach like a stalker, dogged and menacing. There was only one way of easing it a tiny bit, one way I could feel briefly and inadequately closer to her, and that was during the physical labour of writing to her. I knew that all our letters home were vetted before they were sent – ostensibly for grammar though actually for negative sentiment – so some teacher always stood between us, but letter-writing constituted communication of sorts. I had thick writing paper in colours that were inappropriately bright. Forming my wobbly letters across its textured surface with my grownup ink pen, imagining her voice as she sat at the kitchen table in our cottage reading my news and thoughts, I allowed myself the luxury of feeling that she was not so far, even though I knew it was a luxury that was both false and fleeting.

The cliché dictates that food should have been the place I looked for comfort, that therein lay the expected source of solace, but I don't think I turned to it particularly. The hunger and nausea I felt remained unrelieved by Mrs McCombie's baked beans with added butter and chocolate semolina. I didn't eat unusual amounts of either. Occasionally, when food appeared in the form of the tinned fruit and cans of Nestle's milk for pudding on Saturday lunchtimes, it could be mildly distracting. Nestle's milk was a kind of cream-coloured liquid fudge, a nectar we judged so precious that its appearance would prompt a fierce battle of Bags-I. Bags-I the empty can to clean out, catlike, with fingers and tongue! Bags-I the spoon that was used to serve it! Bags-I the very saucer on which the white and blue can was presented, just in case it had been blessed with a couple of drips during the dishing out (which even if it had were invariably measly and only just worth the licking). There were other distractions, temporary though they were, and nothing to do with food. I liked games of Jacks or French Elastic, watching *Candid Camera*, falling in love with David Bradley in *Kes* during a cinema outing to Salisbury, and writing plays as presents for my mother all about adults' lives complicated by extramarital affairs.

The only other distraction was counting. Counting the weeks, days, hours, minutes, even seconds until an exeat, half-term or the beginning of the holidays. I used to sharpen my pencils and make detailed charts which, due to their seconds column, had the advantage of being able to be continuously crossed off. During lessons or mealtimes I had to lay my charts aside, but coming back to them after-wards meant a positive scurry of crossings out, very cath-artic. When I returned to my charts having forgotten them for a few days, the pleasure of one stroke to cast off almost a whole week was untold. The night before my mother came to pick me up was, in terms of sleep, a write-off.

My mother's jaunty lilac Triumph had given way by the early Seventies to a sporty silver Fiat and the Sixties minidresses to flowing, ankle-length skirts, purple tie-dye T-shirts, short denim jackets, looped earrings the size of a gypsy's and striped, high-heeled espadrilles. She and my best friend's mother were not like the others. For a start they were younger. They had long, straight hair while everybody else's mothers had perms, flesh-coloured tights and skirts and gaits that were stiff. Mine, who since she had sloughed off the shouting second husband and was a single mother with boyfriends, smoked Disc Bleu cigarettes and, alone at our cottage during the week, working, would see barely a soul and eat ratatouille for days on end. When she came to fetch me, the missing would instantaneously disintegrate and into its place would slip neatly pride and elation.

On the journey back home across the Salisbury plains towards Marlborough, and for the gold-dust hours we had together before my return to school, we laughed and laughed and talked and talked and didn't stop. A lot of our chatter was about friends, their stories and struggles. We were trying to recover some of the minute daily ground we should by rights have been having all along. Nicky Birbeck wasn't a close friend, she might even have been in the year above, but she came up in conversation.

'Is she pretty?' my mother asked.

She always liked to know how the girls I talked about looked. If she knew them vaguely she would say, 'Oh, you mean the one with tiny ankles? What I'd do for ankles like hers,' or, 'Isn't it Lucilla who's got the amazing legs?' or, 'Emma Dollar's rather plain and plump, isn't she?' Her powers of observation were unsurpassed. She never missed the most minuscule of tricks. Some may think this means she is impossibly superficial and frivolous and, indeed, when I am cross with her, I think so too. The truth is more generous. Her observations are more funny than cruel. The critical scrutiny – especially of people – might have been inherited from her mother. But mainly it was – and is, I think – part of a more benign relish of the visual world in general, a heightened relish that is entirely her own. For example, I know no one better with whom to go round a gallery. With her, any companion can suddenly see pictures as if they had been partially blind then given sight. She also had – still does – an acute ear for tics of speech and conversation. Both are to do with an absolute passion for detail. Sometimes we would leave a gathering of people and would start to play the observation game devised by Mum, who was always keen to teach me to notice everything. She would say, 'Did you notice anything odd about that man's teeth?' Blank. 'The fourth one from the back on the left was just a shell!' Or, 'I've never seen such a low-slung bottom as that woman's who passed us the biscuits. What colour were her trousers?' Or, 'The man with the square jaw looked like a model on the cover of a knitting pattern. What sort of shoes was he wearing?' I had barely noticed any of these people she had picked out for comment, let alone their physical peccadilloes. Only recently, watching a video of Disney's *The Sword in the Stone* with my three young sons, she came up with a classic, proving her powers of observation had far from dimmed with age. The upturned nose, she said, of the cartoon's hero, a little boy named Wart, was 'just like Victoria Beckham's'! I knew she minded about noses, but this was in a special league and made me cross. It was too ludicrous. It was up there with the times she would put her finger under my nose to raise its troublesome hook two millimetres before standing back to assess it. For weeks after she did this I would go to sleep at night with my thumb uncomfortably pushing up the plinth between my nostrils in the hope that eventually my nose would lift by itself to the required level. No joy. (My friend Lydia told me – we were all of eleven – that if you held your stomach in night and day without stopping it would, after a few weeks, do it on its own and would then remain flat for ever. I was ruthless in my determination and persistence and yet lasted for all of twenty-three minutes. So that didn't work either.) My mother's scrutiny of noses meant that she could spot a nose job a mile off. We differ in that even today when I meet someone I don't see a nose at all, let alone have the expertise to detect whether or not it has been tampered with. A haircut on someone I know, or any stylistic reworking of even a radical kind, passes me by. In terms of observing the details of others I have always been more like my father who – long-standing family joke – once failed to see that the new carer he had just taken on to lift and generally haul him about had himself only half his quota of legs.

My mother, along with her sharp eye, always had very firm ideas about what she saw, what was pretty and what was not. I did not. At that time I had not learnt which attributes were generally acceptable, which were not, and what constituted beauty or ugliness and all that lay in between. I had certainly far from formed my own opinions.

Mum was the leading authority on beauty and lack of it. Brigitte Bardot's incy waist, and lips that pouted long before collagen was an apple in Liz Hurley's eye, were particularly admired but Audrey Hepburn was her tops. Often in the car I would list girls and women, famous or otherwise, and ask for her rating of them. It was a fun game because her views were always strong and I could never second-guess her. Occasionally I would ask about someone who *everyone* else thought pretty, and Mum would surprise me by telling me she wasn't and that was that. I believed her. When she asked me about Nicky Birbeck I had no answer. I had no idea. Next time, I said, I would point Nicky out to her and she would have to tell me what she thought. All I could say at this stage was that she had quite chubby cheeks but that she wasn't fat.

Failure to observe people's teeth and hair, their noses and ankles, did not mean I failed to notice their size. That was information with which I could always furnish my mother. About anyone she cared to ask after. There is a part of me which says this must have been because of my very early concern with food, my precocious worries about my own fat and my unhealthy enthusiasm for bodily comparison with others. And yet I also know that children with no such anxieties rarely let a fat person pass by without making some kind of remark or at least openly staring. It troubles me that I come across it in my own sons, all under seven. I have policies in place to engender no prejudice of fat in them, just as I do to bring about at home the decommissioning of all toy weapons. But I know all my good intentions have come to nothing when I see the boys fashioning AK-47s out of bits of toast and hear them writing off a hapless classmate with a shattering 'fat pig'. It almost leads me – I can't quite let myself believe it entirely – to the unpalatable conclusion that hostility to fat, like a love of guns in young boys and a devotion to Barbie in little girls, is congenital.

There again, abuse of fat people is ubiquitous and children pick up on it. Where changing times have thankfully stepped in to reduce – to some extent at least – the vocabulary and acceptance of racism and sexism, fatism has tragically fallen through the net. Liberal-minded folk who would no more make derogative generalisations about a particular nationality or minority than take to the skies with a flock of pigs, think nothing of casting offensive remarks about fat people.

'I was on the plane back from America,' said one otherwise broad-minded fellow recently. 'Socking great woman, size of a fucking walrus on the seat beside me, invading my space. Didn't have enough elbow room to sniff my own armpits let alone read my paper. Airlines should make people that fat buy two seats, pay *double*.'

Fat people are apparently fair game. I wonder why. Perhaps it is because thinner folk think the fat only have themselves to blame. It seems as if many believe that those *that* lacking in restraint, those whose own self-respect is so manifestly derelict, clearly deserve contempt. Alcoholics and drug addicts are different. We all know that a predisposition to alcohol and drug addiction is genetic and circumstantial. They can't help it and, anyway, if they acquire strawberry noses and wan complexions and hollow eyes these are the symptoms of their illness. None of these things is as physically offensive as fat, which is purely a symptom of greed. Fat people are fat entirely of their own making. They eat too much. So they are asking for it.

As someone who has so long struggled against the tide of my own fat, I find the notion that I am asking for it hard to stomach. The majority of fat people have some but not a lot of choice about their physical state. This is challenging for some to grasp as they nibble piously on an etiolated celery stick or voluntarily leave uneaten food on their plates and see fat people, with what they regard as pornographic abandon, stuffing their faces with chocolate and chips. But, nudge the imagination onwards a jot, why not, and ask who in their right minds would *choose* to be fat? Who would voluntarily invite at best the sneery looks and jokes, at worse the out-and-out abuse? There are people like me who forever battle to be thin and never quite make it, or who do occasionally, but not for long. There are fat people who have stones to lose, not pounds, and whose whole lives are informed by their size and their inability to reduce it. I think of Kaylee in Wyoming, my sister's best friend, in her armchair with her curlers and her catalogues and her wit and warmth and her current weight of 300 pounds and rising. Beneath this wit, which has much of Buffalo Bill country happily reeling, there is her total preoccupation with food (avoidance and bingeing thereof), the anger at herself and the fear that she is massively letting down her beloved husband and teenage sons. Don't anyone dare tell me Kaylee can help it that she's fat. She cannot. And there are fat people who have come to the end of the road, given up the battle and accepted that they are destined to be outsized for life, and that acceptance is either miserable or resigned. Resigned like that of a young woman I saw on a coach the other day, whose vast body drowned a pair of seats, whose wedding ring had sunk into the quicksand of her fleshy finger, who was clutching a large plastic bottle of full-on Coke, and whose each swig was a hearty 'fuck you' to the world. What there are not are any fat people who would otherwise be thin but for the fact they have actively and on purpose set out to become fat. Yes, some film stars of the method school of acting – most famously perhaps, De Niro in *Raging Bull* and Renée Zellweger in *Bridget Jones's Diary* – have piled on the pounds for a role (and lost it all again the moment the cameras stopped rolling). But I will never believe that anyone in the Western world and in these post-post-post Rubens days has become fat by design because they genuinely feel fat is the way forward and that therein beauty, health and happiness lies.

I have a friend who tells me she thinks fat abuse is widespread because the thin think fat people don't mind. Fat people's feelings, after all, are so safely buried beneath skin that is literally thick, how could they ever be hurt? So what we have is a free-for-all. Cries of 'fat bitch' and 'fat cow' rent the air. Even polite people put in their oar. They may not insult fat people, they might just resist being openly judgemental, but they like to comment on weight all the same. It can be especially frustrating for them because while the urge is always there to say *something*, social convention dictates it is only permissible to do so when someone has lost weight, never when they've put it on. So it was, at my fattest and getting fatter, that I'd hear a Tourette's-like, 'Hey, you've lost weight!' when the commentator knew fine well that that was the complete inversion of the truth. They just couldn't help themselves; a remark was going to come out whatever. Even on those rare occasions when I have actually managed to shed a few pounds, I could not relish the more accurate, 'Hey, you've lost weight,' because there was always about it the implication that I had been too fat before and that a reduction was long overdue. The truth is I don't want anyone to remark upon my size ever, with the possible exception of, 'You're too thin,' but I can dream on holding out for that one and, anyway, as the maxim goes and we all know, you never can be.

Fat person walks into a room full of old friends who might not have seen her for a while. A typical greeting from a jovial mate (usually a man, a friend's husband, say) is a thwack on the back accompanied by some sally such as, 'Hi there, big girl. I see you haven't lost your appetite then!'

Fat person in any room in which some food needs to be eaten up or else it will be thrown away. 'Oh,' some scrawny wag will invariably insist, 'give that to [name of fat person]. I'm sure she can help us out. You've got room enough in there for several more helpings, haven't you?'

Fat person, namely me in a fatter phase, having dinner in a restaurant with a few friends. I have never forgotten it. I was twenty and what is known, horrifically, as 'a big girl'. I was wearing my usual swathes of black (as every day was a Very Fat day in those days, I never wore anything else) and had taken the usual precaution of opening up the large napkin completely so as to cover and conceal my stomach and thighs. Used in conjunction with the table legs and cloth, I could as good as make my lower half disappear. It was added protection from fat stares. We were having that shallow, irresistible conversation that people in their twenties so relish, about famous folk and absent friends – how attractive they were, how good their bodies. (Irresistible to people in their forties too in fact: last night in the pub with my girlfriends we were having pretty much the same conversation, every bit as riveting, as doubtless it will still be when we are in our sixties.) Guy, first boyfriend – of sorts – was sitting beside his new girlfriend. Portia was seventeen and thin and blonde and had spent most of our holiday in France that summer effortlessly naked. She was beautiful (though had my mother met her she might have disputed the nose: possibly a tad too upturned in her book, but not in mine), with flesh the colour of wholewheat pasta, white T-shirt and *hotpants*. The swap Guy had made could never be said to have been surprising. It was predictable. I did not resent it.

He turned to me. 'How do you rate your own body?' he asked suddenly. We had not until that moment ventured anywhere near the dangerous territory of ourselves. He caught me not off-guard – I am never off-guard when it comes to matters of trying to hide the fat on me literally, socially and conversationally (especially with men, who tend to lack the empathy) – but unprepared. In my confusion, fool me, I decided to be open. I would tell them that I thought there was a slim possibility my body could have the makings of a good figure but, crucially, only if I lost weight. My mother always told me I had good legs and ankles. At times I have conceded privately that the thin versions of them might not be too bad if I only ever had what it took to give them that chance.

'I think my body's OK,' I blurted out with uncommon courage, 'and my legs are quite good . . .'

My mistake was not putting the word 'potentially' at the beginning of my sentence. By carelessly leaving it to the end nobody heard it, for the end was swamped by laughter. The laughter of derision and disbelief.

'What?' guffawed Guy. 'Do I detect a little bit of self-delusion? You've many great qualities, Candida, but a good body? Good legs? I'm not sure that those particular two rank amongst them!'

It was a bit of teasing, and teasing's all right, isn't it, because people only tease those for whom they feel affection. When I was three my father used to tease me about my tummy, always done in the spirit of affection, and now this former brief lover who was still a sort of friend was going in for a bit of affectionate banter. I should have been pleased. It proved he remained fond of me.

I haven't seen the film of *The Wizard of Oz* since I was five, and won't ever see it again, but I can still see the good legs of the dead witch, with their red and white striped stockings, sticking out from under the wooden hut. To this day they give me nightmares, as do my own 'good legs' of that night in the restaurant with friends.

A great believer in never taking a penny from her ex-husbands, Mum could not stop work during the school holidays. She sat at her desk at one end of our sitting room, writing; I sat at the other for sometimes three or four hours at a time. I used to play there silently with objects on the tables near the sofa. I gave these objects names and made up conversations for them. Or I drew colourful pictures with my Caran d'Ache felt-tips of families with sixteen children, all with their names and ages neatly written above their heads with a fine black Rotring pen. Alternatively, inspired by Noel Streatfield, Enid Blyton and Mum, I would write stories and plays too. Again, they invariably featured children with huge numbers of siblings. These children were my companions, and that was really the point. I heard their voices loud and clear in my head and could organise things entirely to my liking and so that I felt very much part of their world.

Sometimes Mum and I went to stay with old friends of hers who lived up and down the country, from Scotland to

Cornwall. There was one family we went to visit often. The mother I thought was spirited but could not quite like. Mum was fond of her for reasons I was unable to fathom; old times I guess. She was hard. My mother, though full of admirable determination and resilience, could never be described as hard. Often, when you think things might upset her she says they are water off a duck's back, but that is a survival mechanism; her true nature is softer, thank goodness. This friend of hers, though, had an edginess that was the antithesis of Mum's tenderness and I found it almost frightening. She was sharp both of tongue and body. A well-known cookery writer, she spent whole afternoons preparing and decorating vast plates with pictures made of lobster and various accompaniments, but because she had anorexia, legs like a horse's with baubles for knees, she never ate her own lovingly prepared food or did but threw it all up afterwards. I did not know about eating disorders in those days but I knew there was something funny going on with her. Her face looked disproportionately puffy compared to the rest of her. Certainly, it struck me as enormously unfair that I had to watch her make these elaborate dishes, even help with the laborious task of extracting needles of flesh from unyielding pincers for hours on end, but was never allowed to eat them myself. Such food could not be wasted on children. We were given baked beans. I know I was spoilt but my parents made no such distinctions. I did not like going to stay at her house at all.

The McEwens in the Borders were a different matter entirely. They had a mother who merrily swore like a sailor and laughed till all the bottles of their walk-in drinks cupboard shook; a handsome father who sang romantic or ribald songs and played the guitar in tartan trews by the fire; children who taught me to ride a motorbike in the yard and play on a pinball machine; one son in particular who drove me in a Morris Minor covered in graffiti across the fields and with whom, aged ten, I fell absurdly in love. At their house we stayed up late with the grown-ups, eating delicious dinners and drinking if we wanted to. With the exception of the cookery writer, Mum's friends all seemed to have lots of children and I would almost combust with the pleasure of being in the midst of a huge family, the supreme joy of inclusion made manifest by raucous games of 'He' and an endless stream of in-jokes all of which I was gleefully party to. They welcomed us in and made me feel, if only briefly, that I belonged to something utterly warm, safe, exciting, funny, vivacious and alive.

From five or six, I used to go alone to my father and Sue's house in Staffordshire. It was a draughty farmhouse, its brick the deep red of dried blood, and quite spooky in the top-floor rooms away from the hub of the kitchen and Pop's study. The steamy kitchen had red tiles on the floor, dead pheasants in the larder and a cassette player on the dresser which played vigorously Vivaldi's *Four Seasons*. Pop's study was not formal and imposing as the word might suggest. Sue had ragged the walls in a wishy-washy terracotta colour. There was a very Seventies sofa and armchairs to match which were upholstered in pink and orange stripes. The thin, white cotton curtains were patterned with just a few blowsy brown flowers, each the actual size of a lilypad. On the drinks table was a clear bottle of *Mar de Viper*, a brandy given to my father on a trip to France. It amused him to keep it on show. It never failed to give visitors a fright because inside it was a real dead snake. It had been put into the bottle alive and, as it had drowned, had released its own venom. The resulting liqueur was meant to do wonders for the menstruating girls and achy old women of Lyons. I was too chicken ever to try it but Pop did once and said it tasted of bird's nest. Above the fireplace was a painting of the back view of a reclining nude by Tony Fry. From a young age it struck me as a thing of astounding colour and beauty, not least because I admired so much the figure's sharply defined bum and hip as they sank into a waist that was elegant and trim. Beneath it, and in front of the fire which exercised a lot of Pop's time, expertise and patience, Sue and I would set up the blue-felt card table and have games of Pelmanism (until I began to beat Pop), 'Vingt et Un' and 'Racing Demon'. Taught 'Racing Demon' by her aunt who had been champion of all England, Sue was a brilliant and exhilarating player. Pop could not be quick, the muscles saw to that, but he had the benefit of cunning. He and I loved playing but against Sue we had not got a hope. It was with exhaustion and spent nerves that after a few games we exchanged the cards for plates and ate our supper of scrambled eggs on toast beside the embers.

At weekends he and she often had family and friends to stay. Netherset was, with Sue's cooking and vitality and Pop's irresistible company, a good pit-stop for those travelling between North and South. Their friends ranged from a bonkers ecologist who wore ankle-length multicoloured dreamcoats in silk to an archaeologist who rolled joints all day and all night. Sometimes he enlisted my help. He would crumble the dope and I would sprinkle it over the Rizla paper and tobacco. There was light dope and dark dope. When I asked him if it was like salt and pepper for cigarettes he told me that that was the perfect description and I felt pleased because he was also a poet and my father did not go in much for compliments. I think Pop wanted to compensate for my mother whom he felt, in terms of compliments and demonstrative love, went way overboard.

When Nathaniel and Charity were born I busied around them with bottles and nappies, a good outlet for my bossiness. Although I was thrilled to have more half-siblings, they were seven or eight years younger than me so did not really come into their own as companions till later. I still spent a lot of time on my own playing in haylofts in the farm buildings, making dens in the bales, stroking the wet noses of big-eyed calves in their pens and wading in wellington boots across the yard to the milk parlour through the sloppy green carpet of cowshit. Watching the heifers loping with weary resignation into the cold, neon-lit concrete spaces by the milking machines to have their undignified udders yanked this way and that was always diverting, as was peering into the vast steel tank into which their milk spurted and I was tempted to dive. On the wall by the tank was a notebook with the grubbiest pages you ever saw and a biro hanging on the kind of frayed blue plastic string used for tying up fertiliser sacks and straw. Next to the pad sat an old black bakelite telephone strictly for the farmer's use only. Sometimes, because my father never liked me to linger in private or at any length on his telephone having what he considered to be sentimental or 'soppy' conversations with my mother, I would risk the farmer's wrath and ring her from the farm one. They were invariably tense calls. I could barely hear her because of the oceanic whoosh of milk by my side and I was terrified that the farmer would walk in any minute and chivy me with the fat wand he used to shoo cows in from the fields. Occasionally the frustration of hearing the timbre of her voice but not her words would make me cry. I would go inside, up to my room on the top floor, lie on my bed and, full of self-pity, read *Charlotte's Web*, which was unbearably sad and only made matters worse.

A bit of a backseat driver, my father used to direct Sue when she cooked but he was crap at it himself. Sometimes she threw a saucepan at him and who can blame her? I think she was once moved to box an ear and he only discovered the drum was broken when he lit a cigarette and smoke drifted out of the wrong orifice. He was on shaky ground. I remember him telling me to warm up some baked beans. I went to the kitchen, opened the tin and poured them into the saucepan but, being five and uncertain about such things, did not know how high to put the flame beneath it. Frightened, I ran back to his study to ask him.

'Don't be so *stupid*,' he balled at me. 'You just boil a pan of water and *put the tin in*!'

Sue, with or without his interference, became a seriously good cook. In the mid-Seventies Pop was commissioned to write a book called *The Great Chefs of France*, which meant he had to go on a gastronomic epic to interview all the Michelin three star restaurateurs outside Paris — of which there were thirteen at the time. (Despite his relish of good food my father was not a greedy man. He struggled to eat six-course lunches and dinners every day for two months and quite often sneaked what he could not manage on to the plate of his more robust companion. Also to his aid came an excellent pill the size of a horse drench. It was called Festale and made of ox bile. One a day apparently made it possible to eat twice as much and was something I often wished I could have laid my hands on later in life when I was gripped by the pain of a bulimic binge.) I asked him what made their food so superior. I could not think for all the world that food could come better than Mum's blackberry and apple crumble or Sue's roast chicken and bread sauce. He explained that these famed chefs created dishes beyond my imagination and showed me the book's photographs with *un filet de loup au caviar* here, *lapin en gêlée* there, and *foie gras* – which demanded a full explanation, the stuffing of wretched geese and all – sculpted to look like a hedgehog with truffles for eyes. When I saw these pictures for the first time *my* eyes popped out of my head. I thought, thank God I was too young to accompany him on one of his grand French tours. If I had, it would have been me who turned into *foie gras* never mind so many hapless geese.

Back with Mum, most holidays we used to drive from Wiltshire to the New Forest for a few days' stay at Ipley, the not-pretty house (according to my mother – her acute eye extends to inanimate objects as well as animate ones) which belonged to her sister, Trish, and Trish's first husband, Richard. Trish's welcoming kisses landing high on your cheeks were so high-pitched that you feared for your eardrums but forgave her because of their sheer enthusiasm. One Christmas Day we spied a cow in a field chewing the cud with the saddest expression you ever saw. When Mum remarked that this cow didn't look as if she was having a very happy Christmas, Trish laughed till she literally peed in her pants. Her humour is part of her charm, as is her singular style of dress (to which she adheres to this day) – Victorian-look ankle boots, long corduroy skirts, wide belts, white shirts with high, frilled collars and embroidered bolero jackets. This ensemble was quite a statement in the Seventies and reminded Mum, she always said, of the town square dancers in the first scene of a pantomime.

Trish, eighteen months younger than my mother, was, and remains, a very different creature from her. Mum is someone for whom youth was the thing. It was never wasted on her. It bestowed upon her an amazing energy and vivacity which along with her beauty was a potent mix. She liked walking into rooms and turning a head or two. She liked the boy-friends that these beguiling qualities effortlessly engendered. She has been happily married to my second stepfather for twenty-seven years so has long had no need of boyfriends but growing older – she is now sixty-six – has nonetheless been a hideous ordeal, as it must be for many whose looks have served them well. The pile of books beside the loo in her bathroom are all about combating wrinkles, the extortionate pots on her dressing table full of the cosmetic equivalent of the emperor's new clothes: creams promising anti-aging properties cynically designed for the deluded. Sometimes I catch her in her mirror, forefingers pushing her cheeks and chin upwards and back, trying to recapture the past with a butterfly net. Her fantasies are of face-lifts. Yet she would never have one because her rational self would not approve, would consider it vain, self-indulgent, extravagant and, in the end, pointless. Her diet, undertaken as a teenager and grittily maintained ever since, has worked all her life despite her habit of solitarily picking at leftovers in the larder (lots of tell-tale chewing when she reappears in the kitchen). But these days she bemoans the increasing expanse of her upper arms, her staple celery stick no baton against a ruthless spread. It is a spread which has nothing to do with a waning of will-power, and is anyway modest, but is entirely the fault of the onward march of years. She sees my half-sister, a rave of honed limbs, youth and admirers, and feels at once pride and pleasure, wistfulness and nostalgia.

Trish, on the other hand, never liked being young. She always had a warmth about her and an affecting laugh that made her presence irresistible. They, more than looks, were her attraction but they were often interrupted by an uncertain temper and an uneasy defiance which made for a youth more troubled than my mother's. Trishpot's early marriage, precipitated by a surprise pregnancy, was to wild, handsome Richard, a property developer who wore tweed plus-fours, commuted daily from Hampshire to his office in Jermyn Street and lined his en suite bathroom with all-over cork tiles. We all loved him but he did have a habit of driving fast into ditches and Trish to distraction. She also had three close-together, spirited daughters (my mother at that point just had me) and a certain volatility of nature. In the past few years Trish has married a quieter husband, an academic, and it has been good riddance to youth ever since. She has discovered with true delight that middle age is her natural habitat. In her Cotswold cottage she basks in it. She and Geoffrey sit by the fire, the odd dignified glass of red wine, reading *Cranford* out loud to each other and discussing moot points raised during sessions at their local poetry course. Middle age becomes her, no anti-wrinkle literature on her shelves. Instead, alongside Mrs Gaskell and Trollope, a banquet of books on miracle weight loss. Perhaps her only regret is that her lifelong diets have never come right for her, and she's done them all – from the one with gruesome milkshakes the colours of dog biscuits to the other where you must mimic the hapless hero in *Cool Hand Luke* by consuming a benumbing battery of boiled eggs. And all the other crackpot regimes in between.

*   *   *

Trish has long been stroppy about cooking. Geoffrey has to eat a reasonable number of sandwiches. This is because after years of marriage to Rich, Trish's relationship with the stove has soured. In the Ipley days she used regularly to have to give dinner parties for his clients of a Saturday evening, the preparation of which exhausted and bored her but she made the effort, if somewhat disgruntled, all the same. She could relax a little when it was just us. Her staple supper for my cousins and I was a deep, sloppy stew, dark brown, with slices of carrot that had gone soft round the edges and turned the dull orange of goldfish just glimpsed in the doomy waters of a darkened pond.

Breakfast at Ipley was Weetabix or Country Store – a muesli my cousin Eliza considered far superior to Alpen – with sugar and full milk and, dizzyingly, cream. Boiled eggs and soldiers. But I was always hungry there. Tiffany, Eliza and Jessica were alarming outdoor types. They spent whole days in the garden running and doing somersaults and generally leaping about without ever giving the faintest thought to lunch. They were all thin and brown, of course, and Eliza's hair, which I also coveted, was so bleached by the sun that Trish once got a ticking off from another mother who thought she had used peroxide on a seven-year-old. For weeks on end they seemed to wear nothing but their bathing suits, and often dispensed even with them. Already, by the age of eight, the bathing suit had long established itself as a troublesome item for me. A bathing suit lent almost no refuge for my stomach, and absolutely none for my thighs. I was a leaden, greying dough ball compared to my cousins. If we went swimming I hid under the water, it sparked up my nose and electrocuted my sinuses as I flailed about in the shallow end while they swam all about me like dolphins.

*   *   *

I loved going to Ipley despite the fact it was the first place in which I became aware of feeling I was the fattest person in a room and all that that entails.

To this day to walk into a room with any people in it is for me an exercise – conscious or unconscious – in taking measurements. I cannot settle until I have taken into account where I am in the pecking order of fatness and therefore where I am in the pecking order generally. So it is for the first few moments after entering a room I am like a seamstress on a mission. No one else knows or notices. I do not possess the usual seamstress's measuring tape, the pale blue length of thin, fraying canvas with faded black lines and figures marking inches and centimetres. No, mine is entirely invisible but it can measure inches of fat just the same. I have no pins between my lips – I am talking quite normally – but my eyes are furtively all about me and are pretty accurate at their job. One friend of mine worked in the lingerie department of a department store in Belfast. She told me she became so practised at fitting bras that she quickly got to the point where she could correctly guess a woman's size from twenty paces. Once a customer was wearing three jumpers and a thick winter coat and she still got it right. That's me, nearly, except I'm not in the business of selling underwear and I don't confine my expertise to breasts. I can gauge a stomach or hip or thigh for size no matter how many layers are covering it and can pinpoint someone's Body Mass Index with digital precision, well, not quite.

It is a quick and silent overall measurement I take and not a judgemental one for, to be honest, other people's weight, while intriguing, is never urgent quite like my own. I am doing it to make the critical comparison with myself. And the news is never good. I am always the fattest. In my mind at any rate. Being the fattest doesn't necessarily make me enormous but even to be relatively fat feels too fat. I don't deny that very occasionally there is not much in it. Or very occasionally I happen upon someone who is actually fatter. But they rarely count because they are always men or very, very old, so do not bear assessment, do not really come into my reckoning. If I spot – what seems to me that rarity – a woman who is larger than me, I more often than not see in her a beauty or intelligence or wit or youth which negates her size and still nudges me beneath her, somehow. It is pathetic, isn't it? But this is honestly how my mind works. I wonder if I am not alone.

Naturally no one in the room has any notion that I have been making my ridiculous measurements. In fact, I barely do myself any more. Recently I talked to my friend Raina who is partially sighted. She described what she sees. In the centre of her vision is a constant flashing of neon lights whether or not her eyes are open or closed. It is like a torch permanently shining in the face, lots of colourful, mad dots in its glare, a sort of visual tintinnabulation which her brain has learnt to ignore most of the time otherwise, she says, she would have gone crazy. The idea of the brain cannily affording itself some respite from the symptoms of a condition in order to ward off insanity intrigues me. Of course my foolish measuring cannot be compared with Raina's Macular Degeneration. She is profoundly grateful that when she is concentrating on something else she loses awareness of the bedlam of lights in her eyes. I am simply relieved that my fatuous fat awareness is a lot of the time on automatic pilot, my brain thoughtfully working to ensure I don't even notice it. I am lucky too that I do not necessarily recognise, with the measuring results just in, the adjustments I make to my behaviour, but adjustments I invariably make.

It is a sorry truth that once I have gathered that I am the fattest soul in any given place – that is, jolly nearly every-where, with the possible exception of a peanut butter fest in Florida – it affects the way I communicate, the way I move, wear clothes and, it goes without saying, the way I eat. In fact, I developed behaviour appropriate to my physical state long ago, back at Ipley and beyond. My whole character was fashioned out of fat, perceived or otherwise. I have always operated as a fat person, taken for granted certain codes and agendas, just as naturally as I have acted within the goalposts of my gender. Set up long ago, this fat person's personality and behaviour is well-established. So it is that any adjust-ments I now make in how I present myself are mere tweaks determined by my weight of the day and the fat – or, rather, lack of it – of those in whose immediate company I happen to be. It is undoubtedly self-conscious, I am the first to raise my hand to that one, but to be fat is to be self-conscious. The two more than go hand in hand. They are co-dependent.

As the supposedly fattest in any given company I naturally gravitate to the edge of rooms. Nothing I like more than a wall. The security of it is like the security of having long hair (which I have had all my life and still keep though I have long passed the age at which I probably ought). I discovered early that backing up against walls was a simple method of concealing to some extent the abundance of arse with which I have ever had to contend. At my beloved London primary school, after toying with the beetroot too long or jabbering too loudly at lunch, I was once made to stand facing the wall of the long dining hall. I studied at close range the shiny bumps of its surface, colour and appearance of Ambrosia cream rice, and felt only mildly put-out by the punishment. This wall wasn't so bad. Up against it my stomach was hidden, even if at the expense of a bottom on view. I knew it was unrealistic to expect anything to hide every angle of me at once, short of a cardboard box with just my feet and face sticking out. Still, it was whilst serving a sentence up against that particular wall that I realised that walls in general had their functions beyond merely containing floors and holding up ceilings. They hid the whole of one side of me. I have made use of them ever since.

At meetings or parties or playgroups, nowhere to sit, I will always find a piece of spare wall to stand by. Sitting at tables I always want to be with my back against one, not exposed. In the past this was about not giving people the opportunity to shoot looks full of derision or contempt at my outsized back view and old habits die hard. They say gangsters, frightened of being shot from behind, are the same. If I am meeting someone at a café or restaurant I still arrive early to make sure I bag a table at the edge. A place in the middle of the room, perhaps favoured by others as a good spot to be seen, makes for an uneasy time for me. I must resort to less reliable pillars and large indoor pot plants (the *Ficus benjamina* with its dense leaves is quite good) if I am to enjoy myself at all. I exaggerate. With no choice but a table slap in the middle of a large space I do not entirely go to pieces. It ruffles me for a few seconds, I might throw my coat over my chair if it doesn't have an enclosed back, but even on a Very Fat day I usually think, fuck it, forget about it, and get on with life.

I have devised and used other ploys over the years to try to distract people's attention from my size. One I learnt from my father. It was important to him that a wheelchair would in no way hamper his zest for life, his ability to explore continents, cross deserts, befriend people in all sorts of communities, have a life. Knitted into this desire was the ambition to make others forget that he was disabled at all. It was a delicate balance. While he very much wanted his wheelchair to disappear, he certainly didn't want it to take him along with it, but it so often could. Once at an airport check-in a stewardess refused to address my father and directed all her questions at me, a child at the time. He answered each one with patience and dignity but, unmoved, she continued to disregard him and fire the next one at me. Another time, the two of us at a restaurant together, the waiter gave me the wine list. It was as if my father, clearly the elder and clearly more expert than a clueless, teetotal teenager like me, did not exist. Occasionally, though, it could go the other way. One triumphant moment was when a couple who had never met him, friends of friends, turned up for lunch at the house in France where he lived for a time. A great raconteur, he delighted them with anecdotes and stories, so much so that they entirely forgot he couldn't walk and after lunch suggested they all went on a long walk. They reeled with embarrassment when they realised their gaffe, but he reassured them it was in fact one of the best compliments he could have been paid for it meant they had forgotten about his wheelchair and were treating him normally. It was those who made a fuss who offended him.

He was the master of deflection. Storytelling was his way. I am nothing like as good at telling stories as he was but what I am is nosy and I do like to ask questions. I will ask someone I barely know about their relationship with their great-aunt or for the intimate details of what they do day to day at work.

Amazed and happy that anyone's interested – 'God, no one's ever asked me *that* before!' – off they will go, into themselves, me hanging on to every word, riveted and asking more and more, but all the while becoming gratifying irrelevant. They no longer see me, not my stomach, my hips or my thighs. It's like a crash diet that, for the duration of the conversation at least, works wonders.

The subtext of measurements and the critical analysis of my own shape compared to others, and my love affair with walls, does not prevent me from functioning normally in a room. It is measure, compare, adjust accordingly, all in a matter of moments, and then I get on, for all the world a person able to discuss other matters, relating to the people I have just assessed with no apparent paranoia or abandonment of reason.

It was not ever thus. When at first I knew the feeling of fatness in amongst the thin, it was crucifying. It was the almost tangible, straightforward anguish and humiliation arising from a sense of being automatically a lesser, inferior person. An anguish and humiliation which tugged me from within, dragged me down, so that often I would literally sit on sofas, on the floor, curled up, arms squeezed round my knees, as if feeling cold and trying to keep warm. I formed in my mind the notion that all the thin people were better than me, simply because they were thin. Any positive qualities with which I might have credited myself were buried beneath my blunt layer of flesh. The plumpness, so in-your-face and hard to ignore, obscured all other virtues. I imagined that it alone defined me for others, and that definition necessarily was of a person who was lazy, slovenly, self-indulgent, uncool, one without a legitimate place or voice. Genuine opinions, desires and needs therefore had to be suppressed and kept to myself. In their place I could display only ones that were not really me but which I felt might please others in a way my physical presence never could. I fathomed that to become polite and entirely accommodating might somehow excuse and deflect from it a little. I might be forgiven for being overweight or at least less noticeable. In reality, I was full of thoughts and feelings that were outspoken, wayward and strong but because I felt fat they all had to be funnelled away. Being fat and inferior taught me how to duck dissent and confrontation to a degree that has had lasting effects on every relationship – with family, friends, colleagues, every-one – that I have ever had. With the possible exception of my undeserving mother who, in return for her unconditional love, is the only victim of my truer, nastier self.

I became used to the general feelings of inadequacy and humiliation I harboured everywhere, but at Ipley, when I measured myself against my cousins and their friends, I would recoil more than ever. That Trish was like me and would have paid to die rather than sport a bathing suit, I did not take on board. I never read her figure or thought of her in terms of fat or thin because she was a grown-up. She was just Trish with her screeching laughter and temper and kisses. It would have surprised me if she had ever revealed to me that she worried about being fat. It never occurred to me that adults thought about such things. It never occurred to me that anyone did other than myself.

As my cousins and friends girlishly skipped about the grass I would sit on the sidelines with a towel, praying for the courage to dispense with it. When we went into the kitchen for lunch or tea, I never felt as full as soon as everyone else but used to pretend I had had enough for fear of being revealed to be a pig. I watched food going back into the larder and wondered if later I might dare sneak in and nick enough biscuits to make up the difference. I never did. The shame of being caught would have been worse than the hunger, although there was not much in it.

My next school, eleven to fourteen, was in a town in Wiltshire that had been voted the third smelliest town in England. This was due to a pork-pie factory in its midst. In the summer of 1976 I sat in a circle with other girls on the grass. The excruciating heat and stench of rotten meat made me feel as if we had been attacked by a biological weapon. It made us nauseous of body and mind, lethargic and bitchy and bored. Our game was a truth one, to go round the circle telling each girl what we thought were her good and bad characteristics. When it came to my turn there was a long, long pause. Silence as everyone scratched their heads for inspiration as to my positive points. They were about to give up, but eventually someone piped up, 'I know! Candida has very good diction.'

I made friends at that school who are my best friends to this day but I hated it. I was not good with petty rules devised, it seemed to me, with no obvious logic but just for the sake of sapping our spirits. Or perhaps sapping our spirits was the logic. I felt the anger towards what I considered to be misplaced authority in the pit of my stomach. But I was also a coward so did not openly rebel as much as I would have liked. My rebellion was via quieter, craftier means. I was 'off games', for instance, for the full three years that I lasted there. I'm still not sure how I got away with it. It was a boarding school which, with the exception of a modern chapel made of breeze-blocks and pine pews, and *Starsky and Hutch* on

Saturday nights, had stopped its clock somewhere circa 1935. It took the game of lacrosse seriously. I could not. Instead I passed the time by going on a diet, not such a hardship at that place. The food was pig swill. I remember the porridge on my first day there. It was impossible porridge. For all the world I could not conceive how they made something that grey and lumpy and gluey and filthy out of the innocent oat. What atomic process, what sinister tinkering had they carried out to render it such a travesty of its basic self? I knew porridge from home. In the sanctum of our Wiltshire cottage, my mother used to make us porridge that was more warming than I could imagine any man could be. We used to eat it, in those pre-semi-anything days, with full-fat milk from a local farm's churn, as well as cream and sugar that was pale and soft and brown.

Naturally enough, the cool girls at school were thin and smoked – the two not entirely unrelated. Yasmine didn't smoke but she didn't need to. She managed to be cooler than all the rest without the crutch of a daily packet of Marlboro. This was because she had achieved that holiest of teenage girl holy grails: anorexia. It was riveting to watch as she went about her quiet business of diminishing before our eyes. She started out as a perfectly normal girl, slender of limb and stomach absolutely hard and flat, an entirely different creature from my own, and one which I had admired and envied. As the weeks passed, that stomach tautly sank, like the foil on top of a yoghurt past its use-by date, towards her womb and bladder and backbone, and the very ball of her shoulder and wing of her hipbone began to reveal themselves with the crude starkness of a biological diagram. Her skin appeared to be clinging on to her bones for dear life, especially round her upper arms and jaw. If she smiled, her tortured lips stretched over the rack of her teeth. The following term Yasmine did not return.

But she became a role model and mass dieting ensued. After two to three days most girls went back to the old habits of Mars-bar rustling and prohibited nocturnal spring rolls from the local Chinese takeaway, often polished off the following morning having been inadequately reheated on the lukewarm classroom radiators.

Some made it to week two and then gave out but I decided to carry on. Although I had good friends, I was unhappy at the school, wretchedly homesick. I wanted to be at home with my mother, in our thatched cottage, writing stories, editing newspapers, producing radio programmes on my clunky cassette-recorder, listening to the Osmonds, Melanie – 'I've got a brand new pair of roller-skates' – and Leonard Cohen. I wanted to be helping her to make cheese soufflés, guards puddings (brown breadcrumbs mixed with raspberry jam, steamed, eaten with dams of cream) and banana milk-shakes. Just one more year, she and my father would say, reasonably, then you can go somewhere else for the sixth form. But one year, so fast and furious at forty, is a life sentence at fourteen. Such pragmatism is not the natural bedfellow of the wilful adolescent. The thought of staying at that school for another three whole terms was untenable and yet, despite weeks of pleading, cajoling, begging, my parents would not be swayed.

I considered the traditional tactic of running away but knew it was flawed. Runaways were invariably caught and returned. Not eating, on the other hand, not only caused satisfying weight loss, it also prompted people to sit up and take notice. I had heard about and not forgotten the thirty or so Republican prisoners in Belfast's jail on Crumlin

Road who in 1972 had gone on a mass hunger strike to establish special category status, and their counterpart in an English prison, Frank Stagg, who had died in 1976 having been force-fed following a period of voluntary starvation. These were Bobby Sands's predecessors and became my improbable heroes. What started as a girlish diet, inspired by them, turned into a protest fast. I did not eat food, even though I was made to sit next to the lime-green minidressed headmistress herself, no food at all, for eight days. And on the ninth day I was taken out of that school, never to return.

When American magician David Blaine suspended himself inside a perspex box above the Thames and proceeded not to eat for forty days and forty nights, the crowds turned out to see such a sight. To the anorexic his trick was a doddle. Give or take the odd slice of cucumber or grape or baby rice cake, and the opportunity to sit by a radiator, his dubious achievement wasn't that much more impressive than that of your average sufferer. What was all the fuss, when so many girls are doing pretty well what Blaine did, less the perspex, for months, sometimes years on end? But even to women in general his was not such an amazing feat. For them skipping meal after meal is not so uncommon, indeed for many it is part of their schedule. I'm sure I and several million other women could have told the world a thing or two about not eating.

The press was obsessed and morbidly fascinated by the notion of Blaine's body, after a time, beginning to eat itself. The phrase was used again and again. I don't know if any of them employed the term auto-cannibalism. Probably not. But if ever there was a new notion for Chuck Palahniuk to contend with and with which to shock us all over again, then that is one for sure.

Of course, most of us have never done Blaine's forty days, but I and the estimated ninety per cent of women in the Western world who want to lose weight and who have tried dieting routinely starve ourselves – we miss a meal here, see if we can 'detox' for a day or two there, and we think nothing of it, except maybe pause to give ourselves a pat on the back the longer we manage to do so without capitulating.

Like this massive majority of women, I am not anorexic, I am not bulimic, I am not a compulsive overeater. I am averagely out of control, sometimes, around food. Most of the time I have my stupid, beautiful system in place. It makes me sad. It makes me happy. But in a way I am eating myself.

Incidentally, just because I was interested, I asked Steve Bloom, Professor of Medicine at Imperial College, London, to describe the metabolic process by which a body eats itself, whether it be an anorexic's, a hunger striker's, a magician's or, to a lesser degree, a common or garden woman's such as my own.

When you don't eat, he told me, there's a hierarchy of things you use up. Immediately, overnight, it is the sugar stores, but they don't last long. The next day, if you have no breakfast or lunch, the body starts to break down fat tissue to use as an energy source. The brain switches from using glucose to using ketones. In each fat cell there exists the active machinery for the breakdown of fat and release of ketones. Ketones can be handled in the body. Fat itself, if not broken down into them, becomes like droplets of milk in the blood known as fat emboli. This is something you only see if the fat tissue is traumatised and directly damaged, when someone is beaten up, say, or in a traffic accident, and the fat is simply smashed up. Ketones are what fat turns into. They circulate in the blood and are taken up by the heart, liver, brain and muscle and further broken down to release energy. This is the body eating fat. High levels of ketone switch in after about twelve hours of not eating and cause a condition known as ketosis.

'So the first stage is the use of sugar,' he says, 'then the breakdown of fat. How long fat will last as a source of energy depends on how fat you are in the first place. There is no absolute time, it is a sliding scale. After shall we say forty-eight hours the body begins to lose a little protein. All the normal sort of fat you see on someone's buttocks – the cosmetic fat as opposed to the fat which exists round every cell and which some people don't think of as fat – can take weeks to use up. Only after that has happened does the body move into the third stage and turn with a vengeance on protein as the last remaining energy store. The body will now be in a desperate state. Anything that can be sacrificed will be sacrificed. The person will be emaciated. This is the terminal stage of malnutrition.'

The body is now breaking down its own tissue, such as muscle, which is marginally less vital for survival than heart or brain. (That is why those in concentration camps reached a point at which they could barely walk.) New cells are not being formed and everything slows down. Every bit of the body is getting smaller. The heart is less powerful, the bones thinner (osteoporosis), and the brain slows to the extent that the person cannot concentrate and their attention span and memory no longer function efficiently. The body has to use every cell for nourishment to keep the brain working. So it turns on everything else available including the kidneys and the liver. The cells of the liver in normal circumstances are constantly being destroyed and remade. With lack of food it is this turnover which is arrested. The amino acids that create new cells are being burnt for energy and so no longer exist to perform their crucial task.

'You are eating your own liver,' says Janet Treasure, Professor of Psychiatry at King's College, London. 'I use that image in therapy. It's a shocking idea for my patients with anorexia, especially as many of them are vegetarians.'

'It is not like a pair of teeth gnawing at the liver,' says Professor Bloom, 'but the liver is not regenerating itself. Old cells are dying, no new ones are being formed. Everything is shrinking. Eating yourself is a grim way of describing a programmed use of energy reserves which is essential in evolutionary terms to ensure our survival through regular terms of famine.'

Whether that famine be the biblical or Irish sort, or the chaotic, yo-yoing type of famine that so many normal-abnormal women are voluntarily imposing upon themselves in the contemporary and plentiful Western world.

When still at boarding school and after I left I used to go and stay for the odd night with a friend I had met there. It was at her mum's mansion flat in Earls Court. The gloom of the decor could not detract from the glamour of the family who lived in it. Arabella's older sisters were the two grooviest girls at that horrible school. One had skin permanently the colour of Caramac and a Russian name which only those in the know could correctly pronounce. The other was white-blonde and the first to wear black corduroy 'straights' which hugged the legs so tight that the act of sitting down resulted in the blood supply being cut off at the knee. She spawned a fashion obsession amongst her admirers which had us grabbing every pair of trousers we owned, hacking off long triangles of inside leg and sewing them back up to within an inch of our lives. Of course there were those of us who had the legs for such an unforgiving cut, and those of us who, tragically, did not. Arabella and her sisters were manifestly of the first category. You never saw such linguine legs, such want of hip or of stomach. To sit eating supper at the small table in their sitting room was an ordeal that made lunches at Ipley seem like a picnic.

I can't remember which, but one of the beautiful sisters could eat like a horse because it didn't go anywhere so what did it matter? The other ate like a chick, blessed with an attitude towards food that was at worst indifferent, at best dismissive. Arabella was a well-balanced combination of the two – ate a lot but only when she was hungry. How they went about it was irrelevant because the resulting figures were all the same. I used to sit at their small table feeling wretchedly large. By rights I should not have eaten. Beside them I did not really deserve to but I was embarrassingly hungry and could not resist. To be offered seconds prompted within me a conflict of preposterous proportion: stomach still yearning, yet how could these svelte sisters looking on feel anything but bemusement in the face of such lack of willpower, in the face of such fat?

I was torn. Their mother, Marina, divorced from the girls' father, was in love with Jim, a policeman, and the sheer merriment of their company was infectious. We played word games and charades and gossiped galore and I could not help myself from joining in, embracing it all. I had happy times staying there but eating with them was an ordeal of shame and hunger, envy and regret. It was there I learnt how to eat in front of others – or not, as the case may be.

Lunch

It is not called greedy when thin people eat a lot, it is called lucky. Greed is not greed when there is no fat as its manifest. I remember when I became briefly thinner, I no longer minded if people were amazed at the amounts I could consume. It was so liberating because I knew any comment would be along the lines of, 'Gosh, lucky you, where do you put it all? You must burn it all off, you can eat all that and still keep trim!' Admiration in place of contempt. It is different for those of us who are overweight and sensitive, which I have been a lot of the time. When we are eating with others we must employ various tactics to stave off the disapproving looks and raised eyebrows, real or imagined, which our appetites prompt. Why else do some fat people seem not to eat very much? The maths is hardly just for the top stream. Because we are eating in private, or have developed various canny tricks over the years in order to give the appearance at least of some vestige of restraint.

I am less attentive to these things nowadays but until recently my first rule was always to try not to go first. If someone passed me a large dish of food and asked me to help myself before anyone else, I made coy, overly polite noises and held it towards the person sitting next to me. Before I wised up to the game, my tendency was to plunge in and spoon huge amounts on to my plate only to discover that everybody else after me was bafflingly modest. How the hell did these people manage to be so *not* hungry? What was the matter with them? Did they all have a secret stomach problem? In which case I wanted one too. What was the matter with me? Whatever, it meant my pile of food became shockingly visible, the nutritional equivalent of text daubed with highlighter pen for all to see and NB. I soon learned to see how much pasta or pudding someone else took before me so I, with my indecorous appetite, could gauge what amount was acceptable and stick to the apparent norm.

'No, no, you go first,' people always seemed to say, but I perfected my tone of insistence and they had no choice but to give in.

When it came to my turn, I liked to serve myself rather than to be served. If someone served me they used to say things like, 'Gosh, I've given you too much, I'll give this to Tom instead, I expect you want a smaller one?' How could I say, no, in fact I want this *man's* amount, in fact this will suit me *just fine*? Took a braver person than me. Or else they gave you a piffling helping, wouldn't satisfy a goddamn goldfish, and you were left gawping at your sixteen peas, your chicken drumstick with no more meat on it than a cotton bud, envying other people's plates, which seemed in comparison to heave with boulders of roast potatoes and pools of bread sauce, and wondering what could be the most discreet and least greedy way of asking, perhaps, for just a little bit more? (All those years later, I never did figure that one out.) No, safer to do it oneself. I was well-practised in the art of serving myself in company, ensuring I could feed my greed. During more desperate times, I engaged anyone near me in conversation the better to do so without their looking. I quickly arranged food on my plate in a particular way, fattening dauphinoise potatoes, for example, hidden beneath thinning broccoli or lettuce; slags of ice cream under light little strawberries. The plate was my canvas. I was a food stylist of sorts but my purpose was not so much to make the food look good as to make me look good, so much more virtuous than I really was.

Another way of doing this was not to feed my indecorous appetite with indecorous gusto. I carefully kept tabs on the progress of other plates but like a crooked competitor I was purposefully trying not to win the race. I allowed myself to show polite appreciation but not to be so overhasty, so overenthusiastic as might have given rise to comment. The notion of mopping up a delicious gravy or dressing with swabs of baguette was de trop, one of those pleasures I almost always denied myself. A clean plate had about it a glaring quality. It drew attention to itself like a nudist amongst a crowd of other people who have kept their clothes firmly on. 'Gosh, you *were* hungry. How nice to see quite such a clean plate!' This was negative attention in my book – the implication of course being that I was startlingly greedy – and was to be avoided. So I told myself I must try to leave something on the plate, preferably a good cloud of mashed potato or hail of rice but if not at least a salad leaf, anything. I liked bones – left over from a chicken wing or lamb chop – because even if laid bare of flesh they cluttered a plate and gave a good impression. Happening upon foods I didn't like – a rare occurrence – was a tremendous help because they did not tempt. I put them alongside those ones on my plate which I did like, and found they were easy to leave. The more I could leave the more successful I deemed myself to have been.

It is a truth, if not universally acknowledged, that only men eat second helpings and pudding. Well, that is not entirely true. But in my experience it is a rare woman who does, and usually one of those thin women who can apparently eat such things to no ill effect. (Other thin women are thin precisely because they are so damn good – or certainly a great deal better than me – at *not* eating second helpings and pudding.) Fatter women tend to decline the offer probably, if they are anything like me, because they don't wish to be seen to be indulgent in public. I have never, so far as I can remember, not wanted round two of the main course or pudding because I am full, 'can't manage another thing' or – give me a break – 'just don't feel like it'. I can always manage another thing; I always just bloody well do feel like it. When I decline seconds or pudding it is because gluttony in the overweight is ugly and I am on a mission of resistance to embarrassment.

Progress of sorts: I do eat second helpings and pudding these days without much by your leave, but still can only feel entirely comfortable if others – men don't count, I mean other women – do too. So when someone offers me another spoonful of cottage pie or a slice of treacle tart my answer is that I think I might wait, have a pause. When others talk of needing a pause it is about digesting the first bout of food to allow room for the next. I need no such pause. For me the pause is to determine if others will accept the offer. If they don't, then my pause becomes, 'Actually, I'm all right, thanks.' If they do, it is by way of a green light for me to follow suit.

I used always to say, 'OK, thanks,' when I saw fellow women capitulating, but never without my adding a justification. I don't bother so much now but sometimes it was, 'My diet starts tomorrow,' though I always knew that was a bit lame and rather drew attention to the fact I needed to diet (there was the risk everyone might start nodding their approval). 'Why not, I'm eating for two!' worked up to a point, but only when I was pregnant.

Having plumped for a second helping or pudding – or, 'streuth, a second helping *of* pudding! – the thing was was not to look at the plate as it was doled out. Carry on a conversation while averting the eyes, then it was lack of concentration, rather than greed, which was preventing you from telling the person giving it to you to stop. They could pile seconds on and when they stopped you could look and say, 'Gosh that's masses!' in the full knowledge that they couldn't take your plate away and give it to someone else because it was already yours.

A crowded buffet lunch or supper is, of course, not only a gift for the bulimic but was also a bonus for the likes of myself who loved food, could pack it away like a warthog but didn't particularly want to be found out. You can have as many helpings as you like, it is just a question of moving from person to person about the room, taking on a clean plate and a new load of food with each encounter. It is the same with gatherings at which canapés are on offer. (Incidentally, 'buffets', 'nibbles' and 'eats' – the other two words commonly used for canapés – are further examples of those which my father outlawed. Canapé itself is marginal but French so just about permissible, but 'eats' is beyond the pale.) The only way to resist was not to look at them at all as they were passed round. A glimpse of an adorable eggs Benedict in miniature or a diminutive beef Wellington or chicken satay or neat sushi or tiny sausage glazed in mustard and honey constituted a downfall. You ate one and you ate hundreds, with pauses, over the course of a protracted evening and were never rumbled by others, only by yourself. You could pig out in private in public, if you get my meaning, though these fattening nuggets were usually so small and delicate even large amounts of them were rarely satisfying.

For all the minute monitoring, careful strategies and self-conscious navigation that eating in public entailed then, and still can from time to time if I'm feeling especially tired, vulnerable or anxious, I did not dislike it. Like most people, I could always let go, enjoy the moment, even if I could never entirely lose track of my calorific tally and eating persona. There was a time, blighted by bulimia, that public consumption of food was just too fraught with dangers and humiliations. I was in my twenties and perhaps because I had big – or fat – breasts (comes with the territory; how often do you see a fat person with small – or thin – ones?) and was all in all a 'big girl', I wasn't lacking for invitations to go out with friends and colleagues. Men were possibly taken with the cleavage, thinner women comfortable with the fact there would be someone round them who was bigger than they were – or is that too cynical? Either way, I turned down an awful lot of opportunities to go out if food was likely to come into the equation. (I remember envying the alcoholic. Socially, at any rate, it is permissible to go out and refuse booze, especially in these AA-aware days, even if people might think you're a bit of a killjoy, but it is almost impossible to go out to dinner and eat bugger all. With food, there is a fine line between being coolly restrained and downright rude.) Instead I would sit entrenched in my flat and my solitude, at home with my system of bingeing and starving. When I had bulimia and was out of the easy confines and rigid control of my own environment, I could be possessed to eat and eat and lose all dignity. Better that that sort of possession take place in private.

One of the invitations I do remember accepting was to supper in the dregs of a house belonging to an effete bachelor. I have not forgotten it for two reasons. First, I went home with a regret. He was a man who had a dodgy neck and past and who the next morning disarmed me by clicking out a front tooth which I had failed to notice was false. (My mother would never have been so careless.) Second, a film star was one of the eight people round the table, thin and perfect, and I did not fail to notice she had a struggle on her hands. It came in the form of a large plate with a vast round meringue which had experienced, like the wedding hat of a tipsy, elderly aunt, a certain amount of deflation and slippage. Inside was a swirl of whipped cream bloodied by raspberries. The impression was one of softness and pinkness and the whole beguilingly beckoned. When handed a bowl of it the actress said she could not resist. None of us could. When asked if she wanted more she again said she could not resist. Others, perplexing as ever, resisted breezily. Never one to waste a second's opportunity, I followed the actress's lead appreciatively, knowing that that was my lot, that a third helping would have been out of the question. When we had all finished, our empty bowls and the depleted meringue sat amongst the general detritus of ashtrays, bottles, glasses and red paper napkins twisted and squashed like road kills. Conversation lolled into the night and the actress's eyes flitted to and from the forlorn remains of pudding on its encrusted plate near the host's indifferent elbow. Her eyes followed it when he eventually took it to the galley kitchen and placed it on top of a pile of dirty saucepans and earlier leftovers. I could tell the meringue was still preying on her mind. Then, as the host was handing round coffee, she quietly asked him if there was any pudding left though she knew fine well there was. Could she have some more? A bit surprised, he went next door, fetched her a clean bowl and spoon and gave her some.

And more? He went back to the kitchen to fetch the dish. Putting it in front of her with a theatrical flourish he said, 'Bloody hell, where do you put it all?' I could see her blanch but, good for her, she butched it out and carried on eating. I counted. She had six helpings. I didn't know her from Adam but I knew what was going through her head; it could have been me, and I was with her all the way. In fact, just as the host's eyebrows were about to take off and the other guests were starting to make what they took for witty comments, she finished it. Later, in a quiet corner, I made some reference to the pudding, more one of empathy than ridicule, and she sighed with relief. Then out it came, just as I thought, the familiar story. She told me her thighs had been bothering her (stomach/hips/arse: delete where applicable), she had been on a Diet Coke, chewing gum and cucumber regime for four days, and the sight of that sodding meringue had just made her snap. The humiliation of scoffing in front of everyone had been unspeakable but she hadn't been able to stop herself. I said, join the club. Both in our thirties at the time and with a lot of other more interesting things going on, we were hooked into a conversation about our normal-abnormal existence around food. It was one we both enjoyed immensely, the hilarity at our shared absurdity, and one which made huge inroads into a night which turned out to be so full of regret.

*　　*　　*

It may not sound it but eating with people for a normal-abnormal woman like me can be fun. I am more relaxed than I used to be out for supper at friends' houses or having lunch, say, with those other than what a friend of my mum's calls 'the immediates'. Good times can be had despite the inner tussle with the tarte tatin. The business of watching others eat was vital and serious. Now it is a merrier sport though the findings are no less fascinating.

Contrary to popular belief men don't eat very much, or at least not the ones I've encountered. I can eat your average six-footer *über*-male under the table. I see them toying with thin pasta not much more substantial than a spider's web and failing to finish their modest share of chicken. My husband Donovan is one such man. Bolognese for supper and you can see the glint of plate beneath his weave of spaghetti like the pale skin of a heel beneath a worn sock. My own helping, meanwhile, has more the density of an outsize pan scourer. His taking of sauce is a sheet to my duvet. Afterwards he never wants more and, disappointingly, rarely joins me in chocolate. More often than not he leaves something on his plate. With him that is sure as hell not about some prissy notion of consideration for Mr Manners. It is of course a lot to do with being swayed by in-depth conversation and not being able to do two things at once. (My second stepfather is the same – he can't talk and walk downstairs at the same time let alone talk and *eat*. I, on the other hand, can do just about anything and eat at the same time, just try to stop me.) Men like Donovan and my half-brothers enjoy food well enough. They'll appreciate a delicious dish (another of Pop's dodgy words but what the hell) but won't necessarily finish it and rarely have more. Fit Nat, my thirty-four-year-old younger half-brother, now a kite-surfing instructor living in Australia with his wife and preposterous six-pack – of all bemusing things to his blob of a sister – was once, risibly, a regular chef on TV in Argentina. He is a great cook but he's not much exercised by food. It is fuel, merely. He'll eat something even if it's disgusting just for the fix of calories and when he is satisfied, stop, even if that means leaving just one forkful on his plate. He listens to his mother and sisters discussing our weight and latest diets and raises his eyes. He doesn't get it, same as Donovan and the rest. Donovan had Peter round for supper the other night. Peter's a wiry twenty-three. They were eating spaghetti and I was on the rocket. My plate, a forest of bright green foliage, was very visible beside theirs with their pastel shades of pasta and Parmesan, baguette and butter. The subject of diets came up.

'Can you ever imagine restricting what you *eat*?' Peter asked Donovan in a tone that seemed to suggest that the very concept was freakish and new to him. Then the two of them laughed as if it were some ludicrous invention in a catalogue, like the one I saw the other day for something called the Diet Mirror which promises a new self-image for just £12.99! It talks when you look into it, saying things like, 'Just put the cookie down and back slowly away,' or, '1,2,3,4! Feel the burn . . . 5,6,7,8! Lock the fridge and lose more weight!'

I was in the pub recently, it was about ten in the evening, and my lean friend Nick was urging us to order some food.

'I'm starving,' he said. 'I haven't eaten all day.'

I love it when men say they haven't eaten all day. Their interpretation of having not eaten all day differs from mine and, I suspect, a lot of women's. When I say I haven't eaten all day I tend to mean that not a single morsel has passed my lips since the previous night, not a water biscuit, not a pair of plums, not one bite of my sons' leftover fish fingers, not a goddamn raisin, not jack shit. What I mean is that I have literally just had water, perhaps a can of Diet Coke and at most a stick of sugar-free chewing gum. If you interrogate a man about not having eaten all day – it's a little amusement I afford myself sometimes – another sort of picture will emerge.

'You mean you have had absolutely nothing the whole day?' I asked Nick that night, but it could have been any of the men I know.

'No,' he said, 'I'm starving.'

'But literally nothing?'

'Well, I suppose not *literally* nothing,' he admitted, rather surprised by my probing. 'Now you mention it, I did have a couple of slices of toast for breakfast. Oh, yeah, maybe a Mars bar on the tube and a couple of digestive biscuits in the office mid-morning.'

I didn't bother to ask him to define a couple. That would have been to nit-pick.

'Not a thing since then though,' he added.

'Are you sure?'

'Yes. No. Actually, you're right, I forgot, I went out to lunch. With a colleague. John. What did I have? Errrrm. The steak, that's right. Chips. But that was it. Couple of beers. Cheese maybe. Yes, cheese. A delicious Cheddar, actually. Or was it Stilton?'

'No pudding?'

'No.'

'Anyway, nothing since lunch?'

'Right. My secretary was handing round some of her daughter's wedding cake this afternoon and I didn't have any of that. Only one slice. No wonder I'm starving.'

The four of us studied the blackboard. Unlike Nick I really

had not eaten all day. I had woken up that morning Very Fat Indeed and had been taking urgent remedial action. I had started a diet in earnest, perhaps I should call it a fast, but a few hours later I was now fancying bringing it swiftly to an end. I wanted a starter as well as the wholesome main course of my choice and had already done a spot-check of the puddings. I was looking forward to the sticky toffee pudding though I knew my chances of a partner in crime were pretty slim. My husband is one of those who can take or leave pudding frankly, and Nick's beautiful wife Katharine has an admirable intensity about her which suggests her thoughts are on nobler things.

'I'll have the lasagne,' Nick said.

'You're not having a starter then?' I ventured.

'No.'

'But I thought you were starving?'

'I think one course, don't you?' he said.

Katharine, legs as elegant as those of her lurchers, and Donovan nodded happily. I nodded. Then I ambushed the basket of bread. One of them may have picked at a crust and not bothered to reach for the butter but otherwise they largely ignored it. Imprudently, when my measly main course arrived, I clean-plate finished it.

'That's impressive!' Nick commented and I love Nick, don't get me wrong, but at that precise moment I wanted to clobber him.

Same pub, same situation, a few weeks later, my brother-in-law Paddy said the same thing.

'That's impressive.'

'Little and often', that pious guideline which women are supposed to live by and so often don't, seems to come naturally to men like Nick and Nat with the result that anybody's eating habits which are any more wayward are automatically viewed as 'impressive'. If they think what I ate those nights in the pub was impressive they should see what I can sometimes put away in private.

I said men don't eat very much. Perhaps I should rephrase that and say they don't eat very much all in one sitting, or if they do it never seems to be when I'm looking. I suppose the truth is that there are some men who eat an awful lot but even in these health-conscious times there is not as much social stigma about them enjoying large amounts of food. So we don't necessarily notice when they overdo it. (Certainly I concentrate more on observing women's eating habits although I own that I may be peculiar in that respect.) The ubiquitous assumption, though, that men's appetites are larger than women's is surely out of date and ridiculous. Some are but a lot aren't. The appetite is a wholly individual thing which cannot be pinned down and categorised purely by the physiological needs of its gender. The rulebook, or UK Department of Health Estimated Average Requirements, states that men should be feeding theirs to the tune of 2,550 calories a day and women to the tune of 1,940. Trouble is, my appetite couldn't give a fig for physiological need. It has an impressive history of having been dictated to by other less reliable factors – boredom, greed, defiance, depression, anger, a whole host of emotions. Physiological need fell by the wayside long ago. My stomach, at the mercy of my anarchic appetite, has had practice in accommodating quantities of food way beyond the female, even the male, norm. There is a merry expression for cheers in Russian which, roughly translated, means, 'We will meet under the table.' Forget vodka, the shameful truth is I can eat a man under the table every time.

Day school in Oxford I hated even more, less the home-sickness, than the boarding school I had at last escaped.

When I was twelve my mother met James, the man who was to become her third husband, my second stepfather and the father of my only half-sibling on my mother's side, Eugenie, who is sixteen years my junior. James, an academic, works in Oxford and for that reason, when they married in 1978, they moved there. Following my efficacious fast I was placed in a school near our new house. I was fourteen.

This school was a large redbrick building on the outskirts of the city and had few distinctions unless one counted, which I roundly did not, the fact that Barbara Woodhouse, famous for her bossy way with dogs, was an old girl. The atmosphere and girls at the last school had at least been a bit edgy and spirited and I had made lasting friendships with some of them. Those at this large suburban establishment seemed conventional and dull. The comparison between the two headmistresses said it all. The first wore luminous minidresses with chain-mail belts and clicky high heels and let us watch *Dallas*; the second, a spinster whom it was not hard to guess was a virgin, favoured mid-calf tweeds, high-neck shirts with Wedgwood brooches and flat, lace-up shoes whose very tread seemed to utter the word 'hush'.

For a couple of terms, while the new house was brimming with builders, I lived with my godmother, Felicity, her five daughters, her husband Tim, who was a don, and various other lodgers, cats and dogs. It was the first time I had spent more than a week or so within the organic, heaving bosom of a large family. Their tall house, in a street in north Oxford, was encrusted with a lava from its top to its toe of books which had spilled from every shelf on to the floors, and piles all the way down the stairs of washing waiting to become ironing. It was a house which had Felicity's stencils of grapevines and butterflies friezing the walls, a constant fire, rugs and pet hairs all over the old sofas, bedrooms with brass beds and patchwork covers, and was always full of people. Felicity's third daughter Kitty was my age and a particular friend, and it was with her that I shared a room beneath the eaves and got the giggles. There was a knobbly kitchen table with an old church pew along one side of it, a battered tin lamp hanging over it and an enamel jug in the middle of it with daffodils or cow parsley from the unkempt garden. Felicity always had huge loaves of white bread that might as well have been home-made. Arriving back after school, Kitty and I cut them them into slices as thick as sponges, the better when toasted to absorb butter and jam like so much soap and water. Kit and I and whoever else was around would sit chewing the fat in all senses of the word and not doing our homework. The kettle was in a permanent state of high emotion. I felt I was in the thick of something welcoming and special, that I belonged to a large but contained family in a house with a policy towards anyone else who fancied joining us that was open-door. At Polstead Road people popped in unannounced and I loved that though was not used to it. Mum's and my cottage was off the beaten track, not somewhere to which everyone – with the exception of a few of her more ardent admirers – used to drop by without arranging it beforehand. And, though I would not say my mother was a formal character, she is nonetheless one who feels more comfortable with plans, perhaps because she works from home and is unsettled by the thought of spontaneous visits which have a habit of interrupting her. They were never encouraged. I found the genial chaos and comings and goings at Polstead Road exhilarating. I was never home-sick there. I might have loathed my new school but this household was in my view the perfect homely environment to which to return each day. When the builders had finished at Mum and James's new house and my sojourn in north Oxford was over, my leave-taking was a sad one.

Mum and James – one keen on remote country with only a down and sheep for company, the other more of an urban creature with a library to get to – had found a house in a part of Oxford that constituted a compromise. On the top of a hill a mile from the centre, it had a large garden so Mum could look out on to grass and trees but was only a short bus ride to James's college and the Bodleian. The house, built in the 1880s, has a rather camp tower at one end reminiscent of that on a small Scottish castle. The cottage had been all terracotta rough brick walls in the kitchen with warm tiles on the floor and primroses, bluebells and snowdrops from the orchard untidily arranged in various haphazard mugs and wine-glasses. The new place had tall ceilings, big windows, a lofty hall and wide staircase so my mother was now decorat-ing on a grander scale. The date and spirit of the house called for inherited Chippendale chairs to be recalled from storage, for William Morris on the walls and a superfluity of chintz which even in 1978 was a cloth I was unable to get my head round. It was not what I was used to. I found myself in an area that was decidedly out of the swing and had none of the buzz of west London or even north Oxford. I found myself in a house that I could not equate with home. I missed the intimate feel of the cottage with its creaky wooden chairs that Mum had found in a junk shop for £2 each and were always a degree off comfortable, the feel of its comforting thatch and beams and spiders and uneven floors and plain cotton curtains and three bears' bowls of porridge.

I was cross. Cross with the house; cross I had wound up at a school which was scant substitute for the one I had fought so hard to leave; cross with my mother for marrying again.

Today Mum feels all sorts of guilt about having been a rotten mother to me. She was not a rotten mother. Her circumstances made her job difficult and were themselves rotten at times but she was a steadfastly excellent mother in almost every way. Her downfall was that she was perhaps too good. It is in her nature to be expansively and imaginatively thoughtful and supremely loving and her instinct was to be fiercely protective of me when the chips were down and even when they were not. She always kept at her work with a discipline and determination that inspired awe in my father who erred on the side of procrastination or some might say laziness. Even so she never once missed an appearance in a school play of me as a water baby or the White Rabbit, was never once late to collect me from the gates, never once forgot to take me to the dentist or fill my tuck box. She knew I liked collecting anything with strawberries. One birthday she was away working in New York but sent me a big parcel filled with strawberry soap, a glass and a nightdress each with a strawberry print, strawberry lip salve, pencil rubbers that smelt of strawberries, all manner of all things strawberry. When we were together she would spend hours telling me tales of her riveting childhood and youth, reading and writing me stories, composing songs with me at her piano, showing me how to paint water-colour skies (she had been at art schools in London, Paris and Florence). It was she who revealed to me the secrets of a cheese soufflé or a chocolate biscuit cake, who helped me to understand *Macbeth* and to see the fun in poems such as 'The Jumblies' and the beauty in 'Ode on a Grecian Urn'. All the things, in fact, I beat myself up for not doing with my children. Most of all, despite the period living at Cottesmore Court, despite my going to boarding school at eight, I never doubted for a moment that she was always there really and I was her priority. Her especial guilt is at not having allowed me, despite my pleas, to have become a weekly boarder. This would have meant I could have gone home every weekend as opposed to just for one either side of half-term. Her work often took her abroad and she reasoned it would be worse if I were expecting to see her every weekend then to have been let down on those occasions that she could not make it. At the time I was blind to her logic and urgently upset but one thing was for sure: she was never less than attentive even when we were apart. Long letters and telephone calls were plentiful. So much attention in whatever form possible to the point my father said she was spoiling me. I think that is unjust. It is a fine line between being a good parent, one that makes it clear they are full of love and interest, and the kind who either ignores the child or goes over the top. My father felt she did not strike the right balance though it was easy for him, at a distance, which he was most of the time, to criticise. What was unfair was that all her maternal love and attention backfired on her when it was threatened, and that backfire came from me.

I was jealous of anyone who presumed to step into her and my territory which had been so hard won. Being suspicious and cross, I was surly with the boyfriends between her second and third marriages and foul to James in particular, rude, unkind and openly insulting for several years. In return he was tolerant, kind and generous. Any lesser man, however much he loved my mother, would have regarded me as some kind of malign poltergeist and made his excuses. As it was James not only married Mum but, twenty-eight years after meeting me, denies all knowledge of my having behaved in a manner that was anything short of delightful. It is a magnanimous form of amnesia he has.

It was comforting not to be boarding, to be close to my mum after years of yearning deep in the stomach for her presence, but I suppose I regretted my move. At the new school and living in the house on the hill I felt cut off from old friends, from fun and from action. Bicycling up the steep hill back from north Oxford or the centre was too much like hard work and Mum was strict about homework so I did not go out much to meet up with friends. Instead I took to running up Mum's telephone bills with a lot of idle chat and watching a great deal of television. Episodes of *Brideshead Revisited* and *The Jewel in the Crown* were as eagerly anticipated by me as parties were by my peers. Sad. Various cousins and old friends were finishing exams, making it to Oxford or other universities or living in London, all of them endlessly clubbing and going to gigs and having various sexual grapplings which were giving rise to enviably complicated emotions. Meanwhile I plumply sat about in our rather underpopulated house with a furious sense of Missing Out and Not Belonging, all the while studying my navel and finding it wanting.

I suppose the History, English and French lessons at school were mildly diverting, as well as Russian with an octogenarian tutor near Polstead Road who had loved the Revolution because it had meant she could obtain cheap tickets to the Kirov and felt for the first time pangs of real hunger, which she described to me lyrically and told me she had found inspiring. But during Maths and Chemistry my concentration was otherwise engaged, raging that I was not in London in all the right places enjoying nights out with friends and callous romances with breezy youths. Between classes I spent my time avoiding PE and thinking and talking a great deal about diets and illicitly comparing my thighs to Julia's. Julia's legs were quite something to behold in a gym skirt and, the way I saw it, landed her no end of boyfriends (and later, I heard, an advantageous husband). I was belligerent and cross but at least at that school I did not have to contend with the food. It was so particularly foul and home was so conveniently close that I wandered back there for lunch each day. As I lolloped up the hill I wished I still had a cause crucial enough to give me the strength afresh to starve. My desire to be thin had not waned but since starting the new school I had simply lost the knack. I ate nothing all day then would have thick, buttered brown toast for tea with soft brown sugar and cinnamon on top, still bubbling bumptiously from under the grill. You can't argue with that. (My beloved second stepfather is one of those curious people, lean as a bean, who faints with hunger if he doesn't eat every three hours. So it was that old-fashioned afternoon tea – muffins, crumpets, gingernut biscuits and coffee cake or, lordy, *lardy* cake at 5,000 calories a slice – became a necessary feature in our house and one which I could do little to resist.) I would start a 'sensible' diet. The Mayo Clinic one, the Atkins of its time, advocated a sulphurous *nine* boiled eggs to be eaten on the first day. I made it to day four, weighed myself, had put on two pounds and thought, fuck this for a laugh. I was back on Mum's puddings before you could say 'tablespoon'. Then I decided on a particular type of cracker for lunch: a yellowing polystyrene rectangle reminiscent of an orthopaedic mattress designed for a hamster was the way forward. It was new on the scene and evidently the pride of its manufacturer's marketing department. My mum and I were taken in and thought they were a revelation. You can still buy them. They are eighteen calories a piece and constitute the nutritional equivalent of a magic trick. You put them on your tongue, you bite and even hear a crunch, but there is nothing there; they taste of thin air. You could eat ninety-seven of the damn things and still have no need to loosen your belt. In the picture on the packet they are decorated with an inert-looking glob of cottage cheese, a slice of very orange tomato and a frivolous frill of lettuce. You get the point. There is no point. Even a socking great layer of peanut butter and jam could not save those mimsy crackers. Naturally enough, they did not remain my way forward for long.

From those days to this I have had an aloof relationship with lunch. I do eat it every so often, usually when I go back to Oxford and Mum produces beef that is pink in the middle with crunchy roast potatoes, Yorkshire pudding and chocolate soufflés that are my undoing. But no one claims that it is the most important meal of the day, as they do with breakfast, ergo it seems reasonable on the whole to make do without it. I think quite a lot of other women feel the same. Especially when I am alone, I can't be bothered with it and am pleased for the saving on calories. On a weekday I might have an apple and banana at my desk, or a couple of rice cakes, certainly never anything as decadent as a sandwich engorged with bacon, avocado and mayonnaise; at the weekends, even if I have made roast chicken and potatoes for everyone else, at most I have a mango and lychees. My young sons, usually in bed before Donovan and I sit down to our supper, have rarely seen me eat. They went through a stage of calling me Mama Mango. Not good, I know. I console and perhaps delude myself with the fact that they are boys and hope any damage I may be unconsciously inflicting upon them is not as severe as it might have been had they been daughters.

About twice a year I make a plan to meet one friend or another for lunch. We choose a pub or café with good food but we eat little or maybe don't actually eat at all. Strictly what we are doing is meeting at lunch but not for it. I read somewhere that even so-called 'ladies who lunch' do not *lunch* in the ingesting sense of the word. They go to fashionable restaurants and sip sparkly water. They order leaves done up extravagantly with aged balsamic vinegar and see-through shavings of Parmesan and when they arrive note how pretty they are. Then with a fork they prod them a bit this way and that, delicately drooling, but the prodding is really for the sport of rearrangement, as if the ingredients were a set of lacy cushions on a day bed needing to be scattered just so. I don't go out to lunch because the children are at school and I am taking advantage of the quiet in which to get things done. I do not eat much lunch because I have tamed my appetite not to be unleashed till later in the day. I do not eat it because I am generally on my own at that time so there are no questions asked. Lunch is a great deal easier to dodge than dinner.

Recently one of the broadsheet colour supplements ran a feature in which a random group of people had been asked to record in a diary precisely what each of them had consumed for a whole fortnight.

They went something like this: 'Carla, 25, a PA from

Newcastle. Monday. Breakfast: 2 cups of black coffee. 11 a.m. two bites of cereal bar and one small banana; cup of herbal tea as I thought it might help detox from the weekend. Lunch: Diet Pepsi and a McDonald's half-pounder cheeseburger; two dried apricots; packet of chocolate buttons on my desk but I resisted them. Mid-afternoon: half a bag of Walkers crisps; eleven chocolate buttons; three cups of tea each with one sugar. Supper: 2 pints of beer; 3 bowls of Coco-Pops; bite out of boyfriend's battered sausage. Diet starts tomorrow. Tuesday. Breakfast: herbal tea; 1 litre of water. Lunch: 1 cup of hot water with ginger; 1 date with half a walnut. Afternoon: 1 protein bar. Thought about going swimming. Supper: pigged out on a number of home-made flapjacks with my sister and nieces. Late evening: four slices of toast with peanut butter; 1 apple. Diet starts tomorrow.'

On and on the lists read. Over the years I've seen several similar pieces in different publications and always thought they must send most people to sleep. Not me. I read every word down to the last 'half a Milky Bar bought for my three-year-old' and I am glued. The absorbing thing about them is that you realise that none of us does know precisely what somebody else eats throughout each day, even those who live under the same roof. Both the men's and women's choice and tally of food, whether a lot, a little or an 'average' amount (whatever that may be), is riveting, but the women's – for the element of compare and contrast – I find utterly irresistible.

All of us – whether consciously or unconsciously – have designed our own systems of eating (and not eating). It is partly to do, obviously, with personal taste, habit, financial circumstances, cooking skills (or lack thereof) and knowledge of nutrition (or lack thereof), but it is also about feeling safe and in control. The majority of women do not have an eating disorder but that is not to say they don't like to be in control when it comes to food along with the anorexics, the bulimics and the rest. The system which we each design for ourselves is the invisible framework which either confines us – in the case of someone with an eating disorder – or to an extent liberates – in the case of a normal-abnormal person for whom it bestows gentle control alongside the ability to maintain a relatively healthy relationship with food and carefree existence. (In my admittedly limited experience I believe the crock of gold – a totally healthy relationship with food, for a woman at any rate – is a rarity. I have only ever come across a handful who have such a thing. With it comes an unusual freedom which I for one envy the socks off and will almost certainly never achieve.)

One of the things that struck me studying food lists such as the above (and my nosily – for it is quite nosy – sometimes asking people detailed questions as to exactly what they consume) is how so many eat the same things each day. The women particularly fall into patterns, usually of their own devising, which they have arrived at following a process that has evolved over many years. The logic of their eating habits has not necessarily been driven by the desire actively to diet. It is nevertheless often about the creation of boundaries which coincidentally work for them as a way of precluding the dreaded and constant increase of pounds. Even those who aren't very concerned with their weight have in place certain fads which they stick to with varying degrees of rigidity. Most of these systems would seem to insure against the onset of obesity. It might be that their creators have cut out dairy or meat or sugar; they avoid protein and carbohydrate at the same time or, if fashionable followers of Atkins, then carbohydrate all the time; they are the type who doesn't eat breakfast or puddings; they have decided gluten or certain fats don't agree with them; they have turned Mondays into detox days; they won't eat anything other than a particular brand of salad or sandwich or yoghurt for lunch; they have discovered they especially enjoy cooking steamed vegetables and brown rice, most nights; or it is definitely cheese which gives them migraines or dairy products that are entirely responsible for their high cholesterol/eczema/constipation. One of my half-sisters, whose relationship with food and weight is about as straightforward and healthy as it gets, nonetheless has an ongoing saga with wheat. Though she cherishes bread and pasta along with the best of us she mostly avoids it because when she doesn't her stomach swells pregnantly and she would rather it didn't.

For years Louise from Brighton has been telling people she doesn't like chocolate. Bollocks of course, she loves it really, it is just that this line enables her to turn it down more easily. Her partner of eleven years, father of her children, does not know the truth. In fact, she is not even sure of it herself. 'I don't know if I love it any more because I haven't allowed myself the pleasure of eating it for so long,' she says. 'But I remember loving it as a child and everyone loves chocolate, don't they? Occasionally, at Christmas, I might let myself have a tiny bit of the bitterest chocolate on the market because in my head I know that type is mostly cocoa, there's less milk and fat in it. If I'm ever given chocolate, I give it away.' She watches her energetic eight-year-old son tucking into a Mars bar and thinks, that's nice and liberated of you. A Mars bar, and anything like that, are just beyond, she says. My mother and I are the same as Louise. What is it with wretched Mars bars? Mum cuts them into pieces in order to have one slice a day so the whole thing lasts a week. That is how they ate them during the war, she says, so hers is a habit left over from rationing, theoretically. Myself, I haven't eaten one since I was fourteen. There's no need to grapple with and dispel the temptation whenever my eyes hap upon that familiar black wrapper with red and gold writing because there is no temptation. As with Louise, for me, Mars bar temptation has gone over to the other side. The Mars bar is an object which exists only in other people's orbits, and then mainly men's. That is part of the system.

My mother's system with Mars bars is ingenious, but she has a few other good ones besides, which weren't exactly devised – they are not so calculated. More arrived at, almost by default, and they have stayed for the duration. You know how some people say that if they drink alcohol at lunch (red wine a particular culprit), that's curtains to the afternoon? My mother is the same with lunch itself. She doesn't eat it because if she does she cannot keep her eyes open till tea. It's a singular affliction and one which in many ways she resents. Ever since marriage to the troublesome second husband she has been suffering from hypoglycaemia, and this is the cause of her tussles with lunch. It is a genuine condition, low blood-sugar, the opposite to diabetes. She is not a hypochondriac. When I was little, it was vexing for her to have to have endless tests which left her none the wiser but with the problem still remaining: food in the middle of the day makes her impossibly sleepy for the rest of the afternoon. So it is if I ring her at lunch-time and catch her chewing, it is only ever a measly peach or apple or avocado she lays claim to, nothing so nutritious and narcoleptic as mashed potato and a sausage. My mother is not faking her condition to suit her purposes – it is very real and inconvenient and she would do anything to rid herself of it – but it is not unsuited to someone keen to err on the side of slim. The other arrangements which exist for my mother are more wilful. They include a fierce resistance to spending money on food. Generous to the *nth* degree in every other respect, I do not know a human being more so, she does have just one area of economy and that is for almost all things edible. She will give my half-sister and I cashmere bed socks and would give us the sun and the moon if they were hers, but in her fridge is value-pack bacon and pots of yoghurt with bright orange 'reduced' stickers announcing their imminent end. On the shelves are baked beans in tins with give-away blue and white 'value' stripes. Her larder is not so very inviting (many an item still there passed its best-before date sometime in the mid-Nineties). It is a larder much easier to pass over than those stuffed with new organic beetroots still boasting their earth and their roots, shiny poncy pestos in algae green, artichoke hearts broken in simpering olive oil and little brown bottles of Madagascar Bourbon vanilla (£9 a pop) just gagging to be turned into fabulous ice cream. She bemoans the stringiness and expense of organic chicken and knows that their inorganic counterparts are brimming with cowshit and chemicals but she will not waste money on food. There is also her complete, utter and total loathing of cooking, which is a useful stance – or system – because it means whenever she is alone she just won't bother. On her own in the house it is a boiled egg for supper or a salad of watercress, cottage cheese and a banana. Years of marriage has done it to her and her sister Trish and millions of women like them who complain that even in these enlightened days the endless tedious task of thinking up daily menus, shopping for and producing them still falls to themselves and not the men. Ask a lot of women what their eating habits are when solitude is the order of the day and a lot of the time you will find the answer is a bit of this and that, cobbled together in the spirit of limitation and very much wanting in terms of sustenance. The holiday from cooking is one reason, the chance to economise on calories almost certainly another, if unacknowledged. A woman who cooks fanciful dishes for herself alone is an oddity, like her sister who eats out in smart restaurants at a table for one. I admire this type but she is another thing from me entirely. My husband away and it is Special K for supper, several bowlfuls of the stuff, maybe, but Special K all the same. Mum has her old Elizabeth Davids to be sure but, like myself and a host of other non-cooks, she also owns shelf-loads of sumptuous cookery books which remain remarkably gleamy and daily cuts out from papers glittering recipes invariably accompanied by photographs of dishes in full hair and make-up, like Kate Moss, taken beneath £100,000 worth of lighting equipment. These are recipes she loves collecting and drooling over but hates making. She used to be a wonderful cook and still is when she remembers but her sincere hatred of the whole business means she now cannot really face it and wouldn't but for the love of her husband and children.

Puddings though are her exception, both the cooking and the eating thereof, and we are not talking about politically correct little puddings here, your champagne sorbet or microscopic *marjolaine*, without a decent calorie to rub between them, but proper, in-your-face, robust, old-fashioned numbers. My mother is the Queen of Puddings. You name it: guards pudding, Sussex pond pudding, summer pudding, steamed cranberry pudding, chocolate fudge pudding, crème brûlée, ginger cheesecake, clafoutis, steamed marmalade pudding and any number of others besides. People who never eat puddings eat her puddings. They take one look and capitulate, and years later they speak with wistful yearning of a pudding of hers they ate long ago in a tone they might reserve for an old flame for whom they still hold a candle. But puddings are about other people, about the cook giving herself in the sweetest, most calorifically generous way she can to as many appreciative takers at once. The real pleasure is not the act of cooking them but cajoling others into eating them, witnessing their pleasure as they succumb. I think of this as a kind of system, definitely. Many an anorexic knows the vicarious satisfaction of rustling up elaborate fancies for others, watching them eat and all the while perversely denying themselves a morsel, a single demonic kilojoule. My mother is not an anorexic and she does eat her own puddings with pleasure, but I think she would not deny that the pleasure is greater for not being alone in the uptake.

Like the mathematician who sees beauty in his formulas and equations, so prosaic and obscure to the numerical dunce such as myself, I see beauty in these systems. I think of Rosemary from Sheffield, trim and petite, successful in her field, who 'has a thing' about white food. Has a thing, it turns out as we are having dinner together at a literary festival in Deauville, means having a full-blown phobia. We had only met a few hours earlier but I can tell you we made firm friends discussing and laughing about her eccentric eating habits. She can't eat any white food at all. Gives her the complete heebie-jeebies. I remember my son aged one and newly weaned only ever wanting to eat orange food (Bolognese made up a large part of his diet for a good few months), but he was a child and children are fussy as hell, we know all that. But an adult with a white food aversion? What on earth is that about? How in God's name did she come up with that one? She has no idea. In every other respect she's a normal woman in her late forties with grown-up sons and a husband who all love her, who writes good books and worries about her weight. But think about it: no white food effectively eliminates potatoes, rice, cream, cheese, pasta, you name it. There are any number of other idiosyncratic fancies normal-abnormal women have come up with to steady themselves, Louise and myself leaders in the field, but Rosemary is surely up there. I love her system for its total want of logic, its insight into the complexity and dottiness of the human mind. I'm afraid I do see a kind of beauty in it.

In my other life when I'm not dodging raspberry merin-gues, playing the seamstress, yearning for a yashmak and trying to eliminate my stomach from the world while at the same time attempting to lead what passes for a normal existence, I have held down quite a sensible job for the last few years interviewing a different person each week about his or her job. Not your bog-standard accountancy-type job, but jobs like the cat-food taster at Sainsbury's – 'I do, in fact [swallow it]. Why not? The worst thing is the taste, so you're not doing anything worse to yourself by swallowing.' A silica-gel supplier – 'We put "Do Not Eat" on the sachet because people do eat it from time to time. I get mothers saying their children have swallowed them but it's not harmful. The crystals just take a bit of moisture out of you and might make you a bit hot.' The former sugar broker in the City who records vehicle reversing alarms – 'Attention this vehicle is reversing!' – for a manufacturing firm in Blackheath owned by his ex-fag at Haileybury. Paula who daily mops up sick – 'We use a clever sort of cat litter which absorbs it all, then just brush it up' – in a restaurant/bar/nightclub complex in central Newcastle after punters have binged on baltis and booze, and who giggles when she has to call security after catching copulating couples in the toilets. And the fellow from Lechlade who delivers mobile urinal units every Friday and Saturday night to 'designated wet-spots' in the West End and removes them the following morning for return to his Bedfordshire depot and a thorough steam cleaning. These are jobs you cannot believe that people spend their lives doing and loving. The astonishing thing is that not one interviewee that I have ever spoken to has ever said anything other than that they LOVE their job. It is this loving which could make you swing either way – become either profoundly pessimistic or profoundly optimistic about human nature. When I asked Jamie the urinal guy if he loved his job it was, yes, yes, yes. Why? In the split second before he answered even a novelist's imagination could not have dreamed up the reason – 'It's the challenge, isn't it? Rushing into the West End, dropping off the urinals all in the right places at the right time and in time! The sheer adrenaline! Oh, I absolutely love it!' There are some who might despair that a man can find pleasure in such a pursuit but not me. In the same way, there are some who might become depressed by the thought that people everywhere are wasting precious brain space concocting systems of eating which are so plainly barking. Not me. I love it that pleasure can be extracted from such singular sources and that people have secret, complex, idiosyncratic methods – of working, eating, anything – by which they quietly abide and choose to live in order to help them to survive. It is those quirky things, corny though it may be, which give me faith and joy in human nature.

I look at Louise from Brighton who is a lecturer as well as a mother. She is cool and warm and groovy and thin and looks great in trousers that are as no-go to me as Mars bars and bathing suits. We were in a gallery looking at important photographs. We were talking about our eating habits. I don't know Louise very well and hadn't put her down as someone overly neurotic about these things but, as is so often the case with people when the subject is broached, she was startlingly honest and funny about her own history and peculiar ways. She had suffered from anorexia way back, aged fourteen to sixteen, and was well over it now but she still never allows herself any of her beloved chocolate and her partner, Dave, has never noticed in over a decade that she never, but never, eats between meals. He probably thinks she is naturally thin, if he ever thinks about it at all. (I won't say there's no such thing as naturally thin though I am very tempted.) To talk to Louise about food, you realise there is nothing natural about her arrival at a slender appearance at all. She does not have an eating disorder, 'Absolutely not, I'm completely normal, completely, I have three meals a day,' but does admit to a very rigorous system which she employs for no other reason than as a way of regulating desire and fat. She has a friend who is the same though her pattern is very different. The friend takes tiny bites of things, just one bite, and throws the rest away. She does it for the taste, she doesn't want to miss out, but she can't let herself have the whole. If people chance to notice her at it they tell her she is mad; she just tells them she's not hungry and they can't argue with that.

'My own pattern,' says Louise, 'is so definite and strong now that I never transgress. It started when I was sixteen. I became a vegetarian because I was a punk. It began as an animal rights thing but very quickly became nothing to do with that. It was about limiting choices. My kids know I like to eat healthily, and that I like them to do so too. They understand that that is my position but not that in my case it is actually to do with weight. Once in a blue moon I might give in to a Chelsea bun. That is the most bread-like cake there is so to my rationale it is more virtuous than most. The kids just think I don't like sweet things. I eat everything on my plate but no more. My big thing is I don't eat between meals. I eat three meals a day, that proper old-fashioned thing. But if I do get hungry between and give in to that hunger and allow myself a sandwich or apple, the sandwich or apple would become a replacement. It would turn into the meal I would have had later and I would then have to eliminate that next meal, simple, otherwise I'd eat too much.'

The workings of Louise's eating mind are not a mystery to Dave, for he is not even aware of the existence of such workings.

'Perhaps this is down to family economics,' says Louise. 'Traditionally the father and children come first as far as food is concerned. This helps cloud a woman's system. It fits very nicely with her role.'

So it is Dave has never noticed that Louise doesn't eat between meals and has certainly never commented on it. Once – they have been together as I say for eleven years – he told her she likes plain food.

'We can talk about very personal and serious things,' Louise says, 'but not food. Food is quite ritualistic so if you have a system in place it might start to unravel if you opened it up for discussion. I'd hate someone near me saying, "Go on, you can have that, don't be silly, Louise." You might give way. Also, I don't want to get into a situation where I have to defend the system because in the end I'm aware it's my own made-up thing and probably a bit daft, even though I know my food choices are healthy. I don't like people to know quite how much I control things. In the wider world it is better to appear more relaxed and chilled. And at home, very simply, you don't want to have to explain yourself.'

My systems have changed over the years. I have never consciously worked them out, written them down, kept a record of them or explained myself (though I have occasionally been asked to do so by perplexed parents, teachers, friends or partners). Ever since I reached the age at which I could make my own choices with regards to what I put in my mouth, I have done so in my own peculiar ways. At boarding school I had a mind to make my own choices but food was presented as a fait accompli day by day and we had no choice. The only choice available to us was not to eat, and once it properly occurred to us to do so on a grand scale (as opposed merely to avoiding the things that we particularly disliked such as the Spam or geological beetroot and spiriting them into our knickers), it proved a popular and abiding option.

My father despaired of me as a teenager only he despaired of me in quite a different way from most fathers. He thought me a pathetic specimen not because I rebelled but precisely because I did not. Any self-respecting teenager, he felt, had a business to rebel. Those like me who didn't were wet, unimaginative and manifestly wanting in spirit. It depressed him that I did not take up alcohol, for example, although he had encouraged me to do so from the age of ten or twelve.

'Wish you'd bloody drink, get a bit of colour in your cheeks,' he used to say.

But from when I was very young he had spent a lot of

energy drumming into me the absolute necessity in life never to copy others and always to do my own thing. If ever I told him I had done something just because Miranda or Kate or Char had done so he would go 'Pfff' and splutter and tell me that was feeble and sheep-like and there was no excuse. So when it came to alcohol I decided not to pursue it. I had no virtuous agenda – on the handful of occasions I have been drunk in my life I have loved it – it was purely to do with taste. I hated – still do – the taste of all alcohol, even vodka, which people claim has no taste. Patent nonsense: it slaughters a good orange or tomato juice every time. Out of laziness, mainly (economising on unpalatable calories was a bonus but not a motivating factor), I chose not to go through the laborious process of forcing myself to like it despite the fact that all my peers were determinedly making it their business to do so. I thought my father would approve of my decision, passive though it was, not to flow with the tide for the sake of saving face, trying to be cool. I was wrong. He was disappointed that I was missing out on one of life's great pleasures, not getting pissed with the best of them and turning out to be wild and interesting.

Instead I was just a lumpish type, rather prissy, unadventurous and trite of mind. It vexed him that my preoccupations were entirely frivolous and superficial but no more so than it vexed myself. I wonder that my narrow and self-centred view of the world was not to do with my spending too much time on my own at home wishing I was elsewhere. I read French and Russian novels, became wrapped up in them and felt elsewhere, meaning any time, anywhere, would have been preferable.

Whenever I did venture out of my room and further afield I was invariably disappointed with myself for not measuring up. I had a cousin, younger than me, who had endless legs with fishnet tights, black and white miniskirts up to her pelvis and foot-deforming stilettos. She spent truanting days listening to 'Because the Night' and cool nights at the Language Lab. I stood beside her shortly in my long wool socks and cumbersome felt uniform or Laura Ashley sprigs, thought by the Language Lab she meant she was doing extra French, and was not a self-respecting teenager. I was overweight to the tune of a good stone and the extra pounds, distributed for the most part between my kneecaps and waist, informed my very being. My stomach had transformed itself from the hard water melon of my childhood into an altogether more wobbly belly which had nudged itself beneath the undistinguished waist that put in a vague appearance during puberty. If I happened to sit down with no clothes on, my belly would flop on to my lap like a dying runt of a piglet, its body desperately nestling up to its mother for survival. It hid the tops of my thighs. I would glance down and feel the sow's distaste. Briefly in my twenties I had a Scottish boyfriend called Hugo who glamorously sat atop a moor smoking joints for all Britain, writing mystical novels and never getting round to the tedious business of eating. He said that the definition of fat was not being able to see your pubes. I remember thinking that was quite a severe definition. I had heard it was toes. But either way, I seemed to fit the bill.

Resentment at my lot and a mind filled with diets and distant youths I barely knew (who were more or less completely unaware of me) constituted a deflection from my school work. I did almost none so screwed up my exams and failed to gain a place at university. I struck a deal with Mum and James. I would only retake if I could leave home and go to London. I lived in a monastic rented room and was supposed to be revising but continued to spend a lot of my day dreaming about weight loss. I embraced the miracle diet of the moment, namely the F-Plan. The F officially stood for fibre but there are a couple of other four-letter F-words which also would have suited it just fine. All-Bran and baked beans featured strongly. I did not go out much. A fortnight later I gave up both the flatulent diet and the retakes and auditioned for no fewer than five acting schools, including RADA and Central. I was asked to sing a song at Central. Music not being my strong point, I could conjure up none other than 'Daisy Daisy' and then only a severely tuneless rendering of it. I failed to make it into any of these revered institutions and decided on a whim to write a book instead. Because I was not eating breakfast, I spent a good deal of time at my desk trying to pinpoint exactly what I might fancy for lunch. It was not very conducive to progress. I escaped to France and the house into which my father had just moved. It was in the middle of nowhere so the idea was that I might fare a bit better both in terms of work and weight. I remained there for the whole summer and managed to complete a chapter or two. But the sun and the pool and the intense atmosphere created by constant visitors, far from making me more relaxed and therefore diminishing my worries about my size, served only to increase them.

My father, having separated from Sue, travelled for two years around the Sahara. On his return, because Netherset had been sold, he did not have a place to live. Old friends lent him a small house on a beach in Kenya for a few months in which to write the book of his epic desert trip. Then another generous stalwart, one of my godfathers, said he could stay at his place in Haute-Provence for a while. Pop took him at his word and settled there happily for a decade.

The property was on a high, steep ridge overlooking a remote hillside landscape of ragged pastures, olive groves and lavender fields. When my godfather bought the six-teenth-century hamlet forty years ago it was derelict and consisted of about eight, perhaps ten, tiny houses, two up and two down, a few outhouses and a 'street' – more of a path – running between them. His restoration was basic, plain, unpretentious – Provençal tiles on the floors and stairs, cement or brick walls either bare or unfussed by anything more than a casual whitewash. In my father's domain – a couple of the tiny houses knocked into one and specially converted for him – a lift was installed, a few bookshelves, a fretful old hob and a small fridge. He had brought from England some furniture and pictures inherited from Crewe Hall. He found their presence comforting. They included a Queen Anne desk, a lofty portrait of Nell Gwynne and a seventeenth-century Neapolitan painting of Abraham and the Angels. They looked incongruous and magnificent beside the rugged brick and concrete and the fig leaves protruding through the windows. He did too, sitting on his nimble electric chair designed by my godfather in the workshop just a few metres away and wearing his Turnbull and Asser shirts, striped kikoys from Malindi instead of trousers, and Peru-vian woollen slipper-socks. By day he would write a bit on his old Amstrad (with its black screen and green – or was it orange? – letters), or discuss the important business of the day's menus, always with a cup of hardcore coffee to hand. By six o'clock he would be out on the terrace listening to his Hoagy Carmichael or Andrews Sisters with a considerable glass of Pernod or whisky or wine and various companions at his side. He liked to gossip. The subject matter was usually along the lines of other guests' indiscretions. If an improbable pair had got it together the night before, Pop was always the first to know about it. Such facts he gleaned with affront and relish before anyone else because, as he was never at pains to reveal, he had heard them fucking too noisily and been kept awake till dawn. He moaned about such irritants but he was in clover really. Surrounded by his things and children and lovers and pushers and friends and various hangers-on, with his fluent French and the sun outside, he had happily turned his back on England, 'bloody Thatcher and the fucking Falklands,' and this was now where he was at home.

As a concession to the intense summer heat and to popular demand, my godfather, a hater of swimming pools, did build one on the edge of the astonishing view. His original vision that the place should become one mainly in which people could peacefully work did not quite materialise. Perhaps it was just too beautiful and beguiling to remain the preserve of an industrious select few. Numerous writers and artists, designers and inventors did visit but it ended up as a place where one lucky writer in particular lived full-time and huge numbers of family and friends took their holidays at every opportunity.

Because of the amount of visitors and the intrigues they engendered as well as the practicalities of feeding them all, not much work got done. I closed myself away in a studio room in the mornings but the lure of shopping for fruit and vegetables and cheeses and bread in the market towns, the putting together of perfect lunches consisting of local tomatoes and basil and olive oil, baguettes and tomme de chèvre and voluptuous figs from the tree outside Pop's bathroom window, proved impossible to resist. As did the poolside lolling, if somewhat fraught for me, and chat and joints in the heat of the afternoon on secret balconies cooled by overhead vines, and night-times making excessive merry. It was a paradise of sorts but one not wanting in its fair share of serpents. Neuroses, emotions, anxieties and petty cruelties were heightened there. My relationship with my father at moments looked as though it might disintegrate. He loved to have young people all about him, me included, because he relished vitality, exuberance, a certain decadence and anarchy, but he was irritated by empty-headedness and I was empty-headed. Maybe it was that I overslept on a morning I was supposed to be helping him with his correspondence. Maybe I carelessly knocked his bad ankle as his pusher or when I lifted him out of the bath. Maybe it was that I invited eight friends for three nights without asking him or revealed myself to be terminally stupid by not knowing a basic historical fact or fancied myself as a rather better French speaker than I was. He could not abide in me a certain level of selfishness, what he saw as an abhorrent and inexcusable ignorance (despite an expensive education) and an unforgivable triteness of outlook and mind. We had great moments of intimacy, understanding and laughter and he surprised me sometimes with unexpected compliments – 'You were clever not to get lost on the way to Cavaillon,' or, 'You're looking pretty today' – not a usual part of his paternal lexicon. One day he said in conversation that if he discovered I was not his biological daughter (I am), it would not make any difference to the way he felt about me, it would not mean he would love me one jot less. He confided in me (not least about his emotional life, which was varied) and enjoyed my company because he loved me but, bottom line, when I was nineteen, I disappointed him. Knowledge, quirkiness, beauty and broad-mindedness were the qualities he admired in someone. He just could not, then, think of me as very interesting or appealing. I minded massively and tried to please, which only made matters worse. He had a cruel streak and a habit during lunch of making his irritation known in public so I felt diminished in all but size.

By the pool my body had a way of growing more inadequate by the day. The other girls, for whom even a derisory bikini was superfluous, were invariably made up mostly of limb and self-assurance and I was not, and their male counterparts were clearly full of giddy appreciation of them and not me. Vast towels and Kenyan kikoys were my refuge and defence, though even they were unable to contain my body's overflowing flesh. I smothered myself in them and sweated. I had no need of Hawaiian Tropic, the dark runny oil smelling of coconuts that they favoured to bronze and sultrily smooth over their taut surfaces, because the sun was never going to get much of a look-in with me. But beneath my shrouds I smothered myself in it too, praying that if I couldn't look as good as all the rest then maybe I could try and smell as nice at least.

I loved that place, curiously, though, because I learnt to hate myself there.

A woman seven years older than me, friend of a friend of one of my godfather's sons, turned up one day and rapidly became my father's new girlfriend. She had left behind a job in a London bookshop to which, after a few days of her two-week holiday, it became evident she was not going to return. There was a vacancy and I had the scoop. After three months of too little work and too much indulgence, I was the taker. It was a one-room independent general bookshop in

141

the West End owned by a flamboyant publisher. I returned to London to take up the post of salesgirl alongside Stephen, the fogeyish manager.

I lived alone in a basement flat with a view on to a brick wall. It was so small my double bed took up the entire bedroom and in the sitting room there was no space for a table. If a friend came round we had to sit on the sofa to eat from our laps, our knees touching the telly. I could not have more than two visitors at once because there would have been nowhere for them to put their legs. But I loved it. I was back on what I considered to be my true home territory, not a million miles from my old primary school, the only school I remember with any affection. I commuted from the flat daily on the tube to Oxford Circus and on to Soho where the shop and the job I so enjoyed was located. Above the shop were the offices of the publishing house to which it belonged but its own door opened directly on to the street. Customers wandered in with a relaxed air and talked about their catholic tastes in literature and their lunch. I got to know and like the regulars, many of whom worked for other small publishers nearby, or for film, video or music companies. We compared our views on various titles and on the local sandwiches and shared a few jokes. The shop was close to Marks and Spencer so I often contributed to the food hall's profits by buying sandwiches, salads, little quiches and cottage cheese with chicken and almonds and other fattening additions. Sometimes, when things were less busy, it was lunch out with a colleague from one of the offices above. There was a lovely Italian café round the corner that did plates of spaghetti carbonara fit for a giant and a girl like me. In the evenings my friend Martha would come round. We would talk about boys

– I used to fall in love with out-of-league or even gay men; it was safer and the yearning gratifyingly tragic – and diets, all the while eating suppers of tortellini with butter and Parmesan followed by full-strength Greek yoghurt gritted with sugar. Weight loss was not on the menu.

I had heard somewhere that black clothes make you look thinner. I have no idea if this is true – it seems to me that only being thinner makes you look thinner – but the dieting was doomed so I thought I would give it a try. I took to black with a vengeance. It was not long before there was not a single hint of colour in my entire wardrobe (although my wardrobe, always scant, never had much of the 'entire' about it), not so much as a fleck. There had been a time, deluded creature that I must have been, when I owned a red and turquoise ra-ra skirt and even a pair of bright pink satin drainpipes (though I admit I don't remember ever wearing them. As a teenager I often bought clothes I wanted to wear but once outside the shop never found the courage to do so). It was the beginning of a black phase that has persisted to this day, bar the odd brown long-sleeved T-shirt, dark grey sweatshirt or navy jumper.

If you are not thin and are anything like me sartorial flourishes in the form of pretty reds and purples, loud yellows and oranges and preposterous pinks, are off limits. In fact anything with a touch of the spectrum about it. The aim is to merge one's physical form into the surroundings as much as possible, never to advertise it. I do not think black does make people look thinner, just darker and so less evident. Of course, a little black dress on a striking woman can make heads turn, can jump-start admirers to sit up and take note. It depends on how it is worn. I have perfected the art of black as blending. The blackened waist of a skirt merged beneath the overgrowth of a capacious black top above. Lines fudged so it is harder to tell where stomach ends and materials begin. Forget little black dress. It is widow's weeds for me.

Opaque black tights are essential. I was wearing these years before they appeared in every hosiery department, when they still barely existed except as specialist dance tights which could only be bought at a small dancewear concession in Selfridges. Pre-Lycra, these tights had a habit of wrinkling at the ankles so I really did look like a Spanish villager whose husband had been dead for half a century. These days you can get every denier known to man, silky-feel versions, ones that claim to warm you up in the cold and cool you down in the warm and, best of all, ones called bodyshapers which cling to you and pull your stomach in a centimetre or two while allowing you, just, still to live. I like the 60 denier bodyshapers. Even 40 denier will not do. My legs require the total blackout that only 60 to 100 dernier can muster. I wear them every day of the year, even during globally warmed Augusts at their hottest, much to any onlookers' consternation. I would rather people thought I was mad to make myself boil so than reveal to the world any of the ample flesh of my all-white legs.

Clothes are of course a perennial problem to someone who feels overweight. I know I am an extreme example of this and there are plenty of normal-abnormal women who love clothes and enjoy buying and wearing all sorts of different and colourful things, but they remain a problem for me. I suppose, along with the fashion industry, I believe that on the whole they hang less well from curves than they do from tauter planes. And because I cannot bring myself to reveal a pound of flesh my sartorial choices are severely limited. Also

I find it hard to find clothes that flatter, to the point that I do not in fact entirely believe in the existence of flattering clothes. What good a 'flattering' skirt if the stomach and bum which it is supposed to be covering are manifestly unflattering? Precious little. So often when I go shopping I see something (black), try it on and it disappoints. Or, rather, I disappoint. If your starting point is an unflattering figure there is nothing much any piece of clothing can do for you. You can forget elegance. The primary aim, then, is concealment, but it is not always easy to find clothes that do the job adequately. No wonder I hate shopping. Rails and rails of merchandise in insane colours and shapes that call for figures so completely removed from mine. Trousers that wouldn't clear my knees and even if they did would make my thighs resemble bellows. Skirts that if the label didn't say otherwise I would mistake for so many bandanas. While other husbands are urging their wives to rein it in, mine begs me to go shopping. He longs to see me out of black and in something new. He has given up trying to buy things for me because while I love his taste and want to wear everything he chooses, I find it too alarming. On those extremely rare occasions I do venture to the high street myself I can feel my pulse racing and invariably come back empty-handed.

My mother and younger half-sister are different. Mum designs her own clothes and even has ideas for them in her sleep. No reader of her novels will be in any doubt as to what her characters are wearing at any point in the narrative. She says she dislikes shopping and fashion but I should say it was more of a love/hate arrangement. Her clothes extend to fill several wardrobes. It is fair to say she does not much care for contemporary fashion; her interest lies more with the singular but elegant fashions of her own devising and those of yesteryear. At her third wedding she went Edwardian, including the waist which two previous marriages and pregnancies had done nothing to unravel. She collects vintage dresses and sometimes gives them to me. In an enduring spirit of hope, she also lends me catalogues and tells me what's new in Jigsaw. Ever-generous, she goes so far as to give me gift vouchers and, if I do get to the shop before they expire, I am afraid I buy yet another all-encompassing black cardigan. She and my half-sister speak highly of Zara and Top Shop and Toast, famous shops in which they find poetry and I have never been. They despair of me. Meanwhile I worry that my gorgeous (another word on the list of those not allowed but what the hell) younger half-sister, perfect in every other respect, may be something of a shopaholic. She is a classicist and a teacher but has found time (and money) enough to collect 493 variants of top. The other night she came to supper and rather rushed it in order not to miss a clothes makeover programme which she called poignant. Two menopausal women who had 'given up' came over all tearful when they looked in the mirror wearing their £2,000 worth of new clothes and said they felt a whole new them. My sister insisted she found it very moving and there were tears in *her* eyes. She and Mum teased me and said they thought they should put me in for the programme. Ha ha ha. It is hard enough to get me into a clothes shop unless one of them frogmarches me across the threshold or I look in my cupboard to find there is literally nothing there and nakedness itself threatens. The few clothes I have are years, years old and mostly much the same. Not long ago, a man who had seen me once too often in one of my tried and tested stalwarts was prompted to say, 'God, Candida, do you *have* any other clothes?' The comforting items I wear day in day out till they fall apart not just at the seams but all over come to pieces. When push comes to shove and I am forced to buy something new it has to be right but will invariably be yet another full-length black tent, a long black polo-neck jersey and even more pairs of mega-denier bodyshapers for me.

Occasionally, on the wind, I hear murmurs that brown or purple or cream is the new black and I am unmoved. Fashion passes me by almost completely. I never buy or look at magazines and pass over the fashion pages in newspapers and colour supplements. Odd times I see how it works, though, for someone in the street or at a party or the school gate. One of my friends who works at *Vogue* always looks fantastic. She has an unshowy elegance and style even on a Tuesday afternoon in a grotty local park with her boys or at supper in my kitchen. Even I recognise and admire it. Personally, though, I do not understand the language. Fashion terrifies me and so I spurn it utterly. I say to myself that it is frivolous and superficial even though I know fine well that there is a lot else that is frivolous and superficial about me and that there are a lot of people who are not frivolous and superficial at all but who nonetheless love fashion.

It is a defensive thing. The fashion industry is infatuated with women who must resemble spaghetti but never eat it. You cannot be fashionable if you feel fat, if you are me. First, fat is itself not fashionable (though from time to time voluptuous makes a sad and short-lived bid). Second, fashionable clothes don't get made bigger than a size 12 so fatties cannot go there even if they want to. If I think about it long enough fashion makes me crazy with anger, what it has done to women. Though I know it defends itself admirably, I with my baggage blame it for a lot of ills. I maintain rightly or wrongly that it has a lot, if not almost everything, to answer for in terms of making women feel shit about themselves, but that is another book. My problem, perhaps. But I feel angry and resentful that it has left me by the wayside and suspect others feels the same. Fashion frightens me because it is like a bully that is keeping beauty and cool all to itself and its gang, and it is genius at making me and God knows how many others feel that we do not belong.

Fashion is most frightening in summer because that is when it is at its most manifest; summer is what it really lives for. Exquisite, extortionate little numbers designed to reveal as much shiny golden flesh as possible, preferably on mythical white sands beside impossibly blue water. Sunny day and warm evening clothes and beach clothes and bathing kit galore. Bikinis in the latest colours and shapes, for Christ's sake. (That fashion can annually wring mileage out of four small triangles of cloth and bestow upon them vigour, temptation and expense anew is testament to its all-powerful hold.)

Summer is my hardest time of year. A hatred of heat goes hand in hand with a residual dislike of the body. In the heat, bodies emerge but not mine. Those of us who do not wish to impose ours on a wider world cannot hide in a T-shirt. I remain in my window's weeds even though it means I sweat like a pig. (Do thin people sweat?) I long for others' abandon but cannot bring myself to dispense with these security blankets. I think there are a lot of people out there who are like me. We love it when cold comes round once more and goose-pimples begin to dust our very marrowbone. When the nights draw in. I have a sort of inverse of Seasonal Affective Disorder, or SAD, a condition which gives rise to depression brought on by autumnal skies and shorter days. My version makes for gloom and misery in the sun and eternal evenings. If I were an animal I would be a mole. Some friends, thinner and more confident, cannot understand it. But my aunt Trish is with me on this. She hunkers down come August in her cool Cotswold cottage and puffs and tuts and anticipates flushes and headaches if she has to go out. There is something dysfunctional about my body, quite apart from my mind, in that the heat makes my head throb and other bits of me swell inconsolably. My fingers and ankles and feet are like tomatoes in boiling water; their skin feels as if it is fit to burst. Knowing that the world is becoming hotter and more sinister every year, a couple of summers ago I installed proper air conditioning in my bedroom so at least I would no longer have need to stifle and crack up in my own house. I hate the summer because I feel there is nowhere to turn to except home, the odd bank and the aisles between the chill cabinets at Tesco. I want the sanctuary of my overcoats and scarves. Our honeymoon was in the Shetland Isles. In January. (It was a winter wedding we had, for obvious reasons, magical dark and cold and candles and fairy lights, perfection itself for me.) I find it troublesome going abroad, with the possible exception of Scandinavia or Iceland, for no other reason than because the heat is of a different order there and completely excruciating. Even the London streets shimmer with a heat that is too much for me and flesh that is so much braver than mine. All that exposure. It is startling. Where do these people find the courage? When I am asked about my sartorial thickness and blackness, I excuse myself with references to depleting ozone layers and skin cancer, all the while scuttling into the shade and smothering my poor children in Australian sun suits and hats or with viscous factor 60 so that they look like melting snowmen.

*   *   *

I worked for the publisher, first in the bookshop and then in the editorial department, for a year or two before giving up. I went freelance and have been self-employed ever since. I had a brief stint in Fleet Street and have occasionally worked on television documentaries. I absolutely loved the camaraderie of working as part of a team all with one goal, the collective tackling of problems, the shared tensions, triumphs and in-jokes. I always liked office life, was fascinated by the politics and even enjoyed the parties. But on the whole my career has taken an entirely solitary course. Times I have felt wistful about this though I have never found a solution because it is in the nature of what I do to be alone. The major benefit has been autonomy, which I prize above everything and which has prevented me from applying for jobs even when I was feeling at my most lonely and tempted. I have been thor-oughly in control of the type of work I choose to do. Apart from my stint at the bookshop, I have never had to ask permission to go to the dentist. I can choose my hours and holidays and do not have to answer to anyone except myself. All this has been invaluable and worth all the insecurity that comes with it. But perhaps both working and living alone offered a little bit too much opportunity for introspection.

Around about the same time I left my job and after eighteen months of living in my basement box I moved to a larger, first-floor flat where I stayed for thirteen years, eight on my own, five with Donovan. It had a minuscule kitchen and bathroom but a big bedroom and big sitting room with an open mezzanine which had a mattress on the floor but lacked height enough for any adult to stand. The ceilings were high and vast; panoramic windows overlooked a wide street with thundering buses at the front and large gardens and trees at the side. The walls I painted the same terracotta colour the kitchen had been at Mum's cottage. Eschewing fashion, I had carpets on the floors, rugs, a mass of cushions on the sofa, thick curtains to the ground. There were bookshelves covering two entire walls, even over the top and down the sides of the door into the bedroom. I picked up some early nineteenth-century French hangings in a flea market. A deep-red velvet and rimmed with small, bell-like silk tassels, they fell round the bed in swathes and were very over the top. Friends teased me that I had made the bedroom look like a bordello. I did not care. It was cosy and a sanctuary, as was the whole flat. Sometimes I had lots of people round, gave them huge sums of drink, and they felt so at home there they often did not want to leave. It wasn't just the booze and the decor. The place had a very special feel of its own, intangible, utterly beguiling and nothing to do with me. Years after having sold it, I still bump into people who remember it with affection and I dream of it often. I think it was this feeling which enabled me to spend hours and days there alone, seeing no one. I found the flat not only enormously comforting and pleasurable but also vital to me. It provided constant succour even if I sometimes felt lonely.

There was no room for a flatmate but there was space enough for worries to abound. One day, when I was twenty-three, my soul mate and partner in regular tortellini and Greek yoghurt suppers announced that she was two weeks into a diet and had already lost several pounds.

I worried I was going to be left behind and wasted no time. I immediately went on a diet too, only this time not one that could be found in any paperback promising spurious miracles but one, instead, of my own devising. I started by clearing my kitchen cupboards of any sign of food and emptying the contents of my fridge into the bin, all except the Diet Coke and unopened bottles of beer or wine which I kept in case of visitors. I weighed myself on Day One and vowed not to do so again lest I should become disheartened by the invariable 'plateau'. This famously kicks in during week two or three of any diet and means you do not lose anything for a while. It is the moment when so many dispirited dieters think, fuck it, pass the Häagen-Dazs. Not standing on the scales was a simple ploy and one which worked brilliantly. (I even thought of writing a diet book which would say, 'Never weigh yourself,' on page one but would otherwise be empty and I envisaged making millions.) I made a deal with myself to do the sensible thing and take up breakfast again, if a very desultory version of it: a few grams of All-Bran with a couple of tablespoons of etiolated milk skimmed of any joy. Lunch: fruit or raw carrots and mush-rooms with cottage cheese, or when I was really pushing the boat out, one glass of chocolate or vanilla Slimfast, a pow-dered milkshake of dubious delight. Supper: a Lean Cuisine and an aspartame lemon, strawberry or chocolate mousse (less expensive, in calorie terms, than a large banana, even if in health terms up there, almost, with the Diet Coke). With Lean Cuisine trusty Findus had developed an innovative line that I considered to be a revelation – a dozen or so suppers (even if they did all taste the same) such as boil-in-a-bag Thai-style-chicken-with-rice-pap or little trays of cheesy-cannelloni-with-spinach-pap to be baked in the oven for just twenty minutes, all at a cost of no more than 200–300 calories a pop. Their polythene and foil packaging with their measly boundaries placed welcome limitations on the greedy dieter. Simply, they made it easier to come to a stop. In the privacy of my own home I used to lick the foil tray clean, but that, if ugly, was allowed. What was not allowed was more.

But there was no more, so that settled that one. And there was nothing in the cupboards to turn to either. So, nothing for it but to shed weight.

I imposed this regime upon myself and created complex rituals for the eating of these identical meals day after day after day, week after week after week. I never went out for fear of placing myself outside the realms of control and losing the will. Occasionally my dieting friend would come round and tell me she had eaten twenty-four calories that day. I felt competitive and the next day would aim for just twenty-three. That was fun. In fact, the whole thing was fun in its screwy sort of way. I liked the hollow feeling in the stomach as I had at primary school but this time because I knew what it meant, that I was losing weight. One evening I sat in the bath and could feel the bones in my bum against its bottom. I loved that. I went swimming and fainted afterwards in the hot shower. I had never fainted in my life. It was wonderful. I was getting results. Then, after a few weeks people began saying I was thin, and a few weeks after that too thin. Yo! No more 'big girl'. I loved every minute of it and what did I think? Too thin, eh? You ain't seen nothing yet.

My family sent me to a doctor. I liked that too. It was also a result, of sorts. He said, 'You have stopped menstruating and are perilously underweight. What is more important to you, the preservation of your fertility or to lose another half-stone?'

Lose another half-stone of course, fool. Was there any contest?

I had landed anorexia but not for very long. When did the strict diet turn into anorexia? It was a strict diet for a few weeks running into months. Towards the end of the diet it became anorexia, for about a fortnight. On a roll, I had reduced the negligible calories still further and my mind and my image of myself had begun distorting itself like a figure in a fairground mirror. Anorexia. But I wasn't very good at it. Perhaps at that point I should have strung myself out of temptation's way above the Thames in a perspex box because after about four weeks of anorexia something snapped. I went to a Chinese takeaway and bought the menu. What followed was a binge of monumental proportions – prawn crackers and sesame prawn toast and spring rolls and chicken and cashew-nut noodles and crispy duck and the rest. The short-lived anorexia had transformed itself in an instant into its less glamorous but very commonplace cousin, bulimia, and was never to return. Bulimia became my constant companion for the next five or six years. Under its malign influence, stuck in a pitiful cycle of starving and bingeing, I successfully obliterated the whole of my mid-to-late twenties; a wasteland in my memory that I will forever regret.

While a proportion of normal-abnormal women are recovering or fully recovered anorexics or bulimics, most have never been anywhere near an eating disorder. It so happens I have but it is important to me not to dwell too long on my past extremes. I do not deny or dismiss them and fully accept that they are behind some of my stranger thought processes and eating habits today. I have already owned up to several daft ideas and fears which I harbour still. Some are commonplace. Others may be more daft than those of other normal-abnormal folk. There again a lot of other normal-abnormal folk have ways which are every bit as odd as mine and more so. I very much class myself in with the normal-abnormal. I am preoccupied by food but my life is not unduly disrupted by it. I am not ill. I no longer have an eating disorder.

The reason I do not want to linger overly much on my own anorexic episode and bulimic phase is not because I am embarrassed (though I am, a bit). It is to do with the fact that the horrors of eating disorders, many much worse than my own, are well-documented. I have read lots of gory personal testimonies. There are numerous articles and books by sufferers who were on the brink of death (four stone and heart only a couple of pumps from stopping). Some reveal how they only just survived. Most have grown up to become mothers and more rounded women (literally), happily holding down jobs and steady relationships, albeit with systems of eating still in place but healthier ones which do not arrest their lives. I cannot and do not intend to add to those. While I think that what goes through the mind of an anorexic or bulimic is interesting, their skewed mindset and the singular way they conduct themselves, I feel that the normal-abnormal woman's existence and belief system is actually more fascinating precisely because it is so normal but abnormal, so widespread and ubiquitous. Almost every woman in the Western world (and increasing numbers in the developing world) has a relationship with food and weight that is, to varying degrees, mildly insane. She is living with a tedious subtext which controls her and her weight to some extent but not to the point where she is prevented from carrying on with the rest of her life. What grips me is that it is part of her ordinary life, and ordinary life when it comes to women and food is absolutely extraordinary.

So to cut a long story relatively short:

The Chinese takeaway binge, first of endless binges of varying sorts, stretched the lining of my stomach so severely that I felt I had been kicked and kicked and kicked in the middle by several pairs of heavy-duty boots and that I was a walking bruise. The abused saliva glands were so sore it hurt to bend my neck or turn my head. Something – more glands? – perplexingly swelled beneath my armpits of all places, so that simply to hang my arms down by my sides was painful. (What possible physiological quirk, I wondered, had given rise to that baffling symptom?) The unbearable quantity of food squashed my lungs so that I was as breathless as a pregnant woman past her due date. I lay down on the bed the better to groan, to contemplate and thoroughly dislike myself.

The outlet might have taken the form of drink or drugs or postnatal depression or panic attacks or obsessive-compulsive disorder, but none of them was really on the cards. Contracting an eating disorder was the coming together of a life's work in anxiety about weight and was, I suppose, inevitable. The only surprise for others, it seemed, was that it had not set in earlier. People used to say to me all the time, 'Gosh, your parents married three times each! With a background like that I'm surprised you're sane or haven't turned into an alcoholic or something.' It seemed to me a peculiar thing to say to someone but plenty did. My upbringing, while a bit chequered, was by no means all bad. In fact, on balance I would say it was pretty damn good and anyway I was never of the school that chequered makes for invariable disaster. Many people whose 'chequered' has been infinitely more so than mine, incorporating neglect, cruelty and abuse and so forth, have come through it OK, without eating disorders or nervous breakdowns or the rest. My stock reply was, thank you, I'm all right Jack. I would laugh and tell people that the shit had not yet hit the fan but maybe they could expect it any day now. When it did I was the one taken most by surprise. At last the joke was on me.

My daily commute was a step through the door between the bedroom and sitting room. When the diet became a victim of its own success I was in the perfect situation for bulimia to take hold and run riot. No one to witness the madness though family and friends knew it was going on. I was unusually open about it because I found the battle between the rational and irrational that was raging in my head and which characterises an eating disorder so intriguing. I couldn't help telling people about it. They tried their very best to make me see sense. But it was a hopeless cause. I saw sense but ignored it. One shrink even said my heightened awareness of my own problem was such that he was rendered completely unable to treat me. So I was able to lock my front door with a binge supply of bread and butter and cheese and chocolate, or not a crumb of anything at all, and carry on and on.

I had an unusual strain of bulimia in as much as I never made myself sick after bingeing. Most bulimics, having gobbled the whole loaf of bread and butter, three tubs of ice cream and two packets of biscuits in one sitting, stick their fingers down their throats afterwards so as to eject as much of it as they can. I have heard how some are careful to consume something like tomato juice at the start of a binge so it can act as a marker. The logic goes that it lies at the bottom of the stomach so when the vomit turns red it shows everything eaten after it has come up. Succeeding in emptying the stomach completely might take an hour, involve any number of finger jabs and a very sore throat. I was never so brave. I have a phobia about vomiting – I have not been sick since I was nine – so made a pretty useless bulimic. My way of compensating for the gorging was instead to starve completely for several days after the event. I was well-practised in the art and it was much less agonising than the enforced vomiting and much less bad for the teeth. (The stomach acids so frequently flowing past in the sick cause erosion so that severe bulimics have only stumps.)

I was despatched to the psychiatric Maudsley Hospital in south London for an assessment and was delighted to have it confirmed that, despite having never made myself throw up, I did have bulimia. It was official. As an outpatient I had to go every week for an appointment with a psychiatrist in the eating disorders unit. I used look forward to my trips on the train to Denmark Hill and his and my discussions about everything I had eaten (I had to write detailed food diaries) and everything I felt. It was interesting talking to an expert. We continued our conversation for a year and I enjoyed it enormously but it did not do any good. I tried a soothing therapist in Maida Vale whose method was massage and chat. I loved my sessions with her. She had a warmth and sympathy about her which made our weekly fifty minutes something very much to look forward to, though the bulimia remained as bullish as ever.

Although it clobbered my social life, it was work as usual. Pragmatism dictated that no amount of illness could possibly interfere with that. I had to earn money regardless of my struggles with food and weight. I carried on doing what I had always done and never missed deadlines. If a work person suggested lunch I would make my excuses and turn it into a morning or afternoon meeting. Only once did work itself fall by the wayside. I turned down a job because it involved going to Cairo for four days and I was too scared of the trip turning into a four-day-long binge.

It was the having fun that suffered. A simple invitation to go out for the evening with friends would put me in a terrible spin of indecision. I used to feel anxious all day, longing to join in yet knowing that to face food in any environment other than my own would be my undoing. More often than not at the last minute the anxiety would get the better of me and I would cancel. I would stay at home alone with my Diet Coke and anger and regret and then like as not go out and buy food for a horrendous binge anyway.

I missed several close friends' weddings. One of my best friends would have been well within her rights to drop me but didn't, and I have felt cross with myself for not going and grateful to her for her understanding ever since. I can think of two couples who have dropped me. I told one lot who were getting married in Scotland that I could not come because my father was in hospital and there was a chance his leg might have to be amputated. It was true there was that risk (luckily it never happened) but my fear of food was the real reason. It took precedence over a long friendship which to my lasting regret is now no more.

When I did go out things were usually as bad as anticipated. Miraculously I found the wherewithal to go to the wedding of another friend, a Register Office affair with just immediate family and best friends. I was not much of a guest. Technically I was there but I was not remotely in spirit. I remember little of the occasion except how I spent the whole time obsessed by the food, how I was going to get as much down me as was possible without the rest of the table thinking I was a werewolf. I went home alone, furious that I had broken my fast, furious that – if you can believe it – I had gone in the first place, and I continued bingeing into a very lonely evening.

Another time, my father back from months travelling abroad, it was arranged that he should meet up with my mother and me for dinner in an Italian restaurant. The three of us together was a rare occurrence at that time and important to me. I summoned up the courage and went but with severe eating rules in place to keep myself under control. The restaurant had white tiles on the floor and reminded me of the ones he and I used to visit alone in his days as a critic, though the food had moved on a little from prawn cocktail and *pollo surpriso*. My father's first comment was that I looked ill and needed feeding up. I looked at the menu and ordered a side dish of vegetables with strict instructions to the waiter to add no butter or olive oil. Pop was livid and cutting in a way that had always terrified me as a child, but I stuck to my guns and absolutely refused to change my order or to cry in front of him aged twenty-five. I had a lump in my throat as rough and heavy as coal. I set my face rigid and prevented myself from blinking, knowing, just as I had aged five, that to do so would release the tears that had gathered on the reddened shelves of my lower lids and the whole edifice would come tumbling after. I told the waiter again that I wanted the side vegetables with no olive oil. When the little plate of baby carrots and mange-tout arrived they were swimming in a thick yellowy-green pool. I knew in my rational mind that they were not so bad really, that in fact they amounted, olive oil and all, to a modest supper unlikely to work untold damage on the hips. But the irrational within was proceeding to beat the shit out of the weaker rational. I began to hallucinate. Before my eyes the innocent vegetables in their malign oil turned into Sendak demons and rose up off the plate to torment me. I panicked and bloody nearly fainted but still would not eat them. I recovered sufficiently to plead with the waiter to take away the demons. He brought me a new side dish, its little vegetables naked of nightmarish oils. A few nights later my father came to stay with me. In the morning I stood in front of my long mirror, checking to see how effectively or not that day's clothes concealed my fat. I collapsed into a heap on the floor. He watched me from the impotence of his wheelchair, shifted his arm along the armrest and upturned his beautiful hand towards me, but despair at the fat I had had to confront in the glass had pinned me to the carpet and would not enable me to reach out to him. He, who had heard about my troubles from my mother but who had long been of the opinion that she was the kind of woman who tended to err on the side of exaggeration, found his anger disintegrate into concern. He told me that I was pretty (paternal bias) and young and doing well in my work and surrounded by loving family and friends and that he was old and crippled (his word) and with a fair few failed marriages behind him, nowhere to live and on income support, but he did not know the meaning of the word depression. What was I on about? Eat and be merry, that was his view. Levelling words indeed but I did not really hear them then or perhaps not listen. It is only now, him dead for six years and my youth quite gone, that I think of them at last.

To be so deaf meant for a desultory existence. I loathed having to turn down opportunities to go to parties and on holidays where all my friends were sure to be having a great time. I knew it made no sense and was such an impossible waste but I persisted in the madness of it for a full five years.

I sat at home alone with a book which listed every food known to man and its calorific value per ounce. I studied it and learnt its tedious tables so before long I could look at any food of any size, shape or form and know precisely how many calories it contained. Friends would marvel at my unusual ability and would occasionally test me but could never catch me out. I suppose it was quite funny but it was also incredibly boring. I became a prize bore, boring myself as well as others to tears, but I couldn't stop it.

While almost every minute of each day I was solitarily, obsessively counting calories, weighing up every pound of my flesh and rotting my brain with mind-numbing, pointless calculations, my contemporaries were busy getting on with life, studying, working, travelling, experimenting, playing, eating, dieting, eating, meeting new people, forging relation-ships, splitting up, getting married, having children, carving out futures. I used to sit at the table in the window of the flat. Friends often told me they spied me there as they walked by or went past on the bus but didn't drop in for fear of disturbing me as I was working. I was working some of the time but I was worrying more. I watched them too, from within the self-imposed confinement of my four walls, coming and going, and longed for a slice of their abandon and vitality. But I suppose I had not totally given up. I did very occasionally go out to a movie with a girlfriend or a drinking club with a few mates (and not drink) and have the odd desultory one- or two-night stand with men I barely knew, sometimes did not even like very much, just for the hell of it and to prove I could.

My old friends were good to me and visited often. They pleaded with me to put my bodily concerns aside but to no avail. Sometimes I made them laugh about my own silliness, the absurdity and detail of my preoccupations, before work or family commitments would call them away again and I was left with the oppression of silent starvation once more.

For a while I had a boyfriend, a painter called Fred, whom I absolutely adored. He was not critical of my figure, in fact he had a relish of the voluptuous and did a series of nude paintings of me. Several of them were exhibited in galleries in the West End and one, at a private view in the summer of 1987, was snapped up by Francis Bacon. If Bacon hated a painting, apparently, he would buy it just in order to destroy it. This one, he told Fred, he bought to hang on his bedroom wall. The rational side of me felt the prestigious sale and destination of the painting might just mean that the figure depicted was not totally abhorrent. But to the irrational side of me it meant jack shit and thereafter I persisted whole-heartedly in my bulimic arrangements.

Another summer, the relationship with the painter having predictably, sadly, gone the way of all flesh, my mother and stepfather found me locked up in my sweltering flat, sun streaming in, all windows closed, with my book of calorie tables in hand, having not seen another soul for days. I was immediately despatched to a grim redbrick treatment centre in the country run by a smarmy doctor based in South Kensington who was more concerned about the profile of his thigh in his tennis shorts, the turn of his calf, the power of his serve and his riches than the miserable patients in his care. (No wonder he was so rich. My six weeks cost the state £22,000, a fact about which to this day I remain guilty and feel was a shameful waste of taxpayers' money.) There were anorexics, bulimics, alcoholics, shopaholics, junkies, gamblers, sex addicts – one with only one leg which gave rise to a few cruel jokes – you name it. They all had eye-popping stories to tell. One bulimic had no teeth left because she made herself sick up to forty times a day; she only had to lean forward, no fingers, and the very motion would activate her hyper-sensitive vomiting reflex. Another told me she lived in a council flat in King's Cross, how she used to steal a lot of food from the station, go back home for a binge and was only able to stop herself from carrying on if she opened every packet in the place, threw all the contents in the bin and then doused the lot in bleach. Only even that didn't always work. Many a time she had gone back to the bin, rinsed the rubbish as best she could and feverishly eaten it all the same. My experiences paled compared to hers. I made friends with her and some of the others but I hated that place with every fat cell in my body. I was not allowed to read a novel or newspaper (a crucial part of the programme, or so I was led to believe but couldn't; a programme entirely devoid of any medical foundation and based wholly on a lot of touchy-feely mumbo-jumbo, or so I saw it). I suppose it was not a complete waste of time. I picked up one or two useful tips from my fellow inmates, such as water-logging – drinking a gallon or so of water before a meal (it was strictly three meals a day, nothing in between and no white flour or sugar) to knock the edge off the appetite and flush any food thoroughly through. I own that the programme helped a lot of people to recover, I could see and respect that, but there were those of us whom it could not touch and who slipped through the net. One morning, encouraged by a charismatic counsellor and the general histrionics of the group atmosphere, and prompted by some insignificant and probably bogus childhood memory, I did have a touchy-feely moment all of my own (I sobbed and it felt mildly cathartic for a few minutes). But other than that I was aware of my huge sense of detachment and even, at times, contempt for the whole set-up. One day we were sent for a stroll along the narrow lanes near the centre and without thinking I picked a perfect warm blackberry from the summer afternoon hedgerow and popped it in my mouth. One of the group saw this travesty of cleanliness – a blackberry consumed between meals, after all, constituted the eating equivalent of falling off the wagon with a two-litre bottle of vodka – and told. Oh, the fuss of the fallout. It was on a par with that which had arisen the week before when the one-legged sex addict had hit on a blonde member of the nursing staff. The place was in an uproar of gossip, consternation and crisis. The sex addict had been out within the hour. I myself was hauled up in front of the authorities and threatened with expulsion with immediate effect. I had never been much good with authority and then was no exception. I looked at the man as if the world had gone mad. And my expression must have given even him pause. A goddamn blackberry. He let me off this time but that was the breaking point for me. For six weeks I had stuck the place out, hoping that, as it had been for others – perhaps more desperate than myself? – it might be my salvation. But no. My future there turned on a blackberry. Time to bail out and head back to London.

Tea

I returned none the wiser, just bitter and furious that misplaced optimism and hope meant I had missed the big day of one of my best friends. It was a special wedding by all accounts, but my desperation had not been able to wait, apparently, and I had gone into treatment just a few days before it. And for what? In order for the solace and recovery I so craved to elude me still at an establishment, in my view, manifestly wanting. My outlook was not so bleak that the fact I had frittered away six precious weeks of life there passed me by. I resented the loss of every single day. When I got home, clutching at straws, desperately trying to cobble together some kind of system of eating to deflect instant relapse, I tried to abide by its prescriptive rules for a while. I continued to cut out white flour and sugar and attended a handful of Overeaters Anonymous meetings in cold and flaky church halls. But I was less than half-hearted. I soon gave up and for a few more months carried on exactly where I had left off before I ever went.

In the end I was lucky. I managed to kick the bulimia habit without any therapist or programme or any other kind of – in my case – less than helpful help. Three factors enabled me finally to get over it.

First, I grew up. I reached the age of twenty-eight; my

friends were progressing in all directions and I was not. I became increasingly of the opinion that it was no longer appropriate to be labouring under the burden of an essentially teenage disorder. It lacked dignity, I felt, still to be distorting the stomach and assaulting the saliva glands with Caramacs and Milky Bars whilst the biological clock was ticking ever further towards its witching hour. You are past the age, I told myself, move on.

Second, I grew just too bored of bulimia (and myself) for it any longer to be tenable as a way to live. On and on it had banged. It had become like a friend who gradually appears more and more irksome and disenchanting till you recognise at last and in a flash that the disadvantages of the friendship outweigh the advantages, and the moment has come to part company. At the beginning, that capricious yet steadfast new friend had not been all bad, despite a few unsavoury habits and vexing ways. She had after all accommodated whim, indulged self-pity, taught one that there were (mainly edible) consolations to be surrendered from the slough of loneliness and – not least – sanctioned the sly delights of gorging on foods that, away from her malign influence, were totally disallowed. No-go pork pies the size of babies' hats, tubs of cookie-dough ice cream and vanilla custard and family packs of Cadbury's Fruit and Nut were just the ticket in her book, the more the merrier; milk-chocolate digestives galore, jammy doughnuts sticky with intent and toast and butter piled like the mattresses in 'The Princess and the Pea'. In her company, I downed quantities of forbidden food at which even Greed would have raised an eyebrow and viewed as immodest, and I enjoyed it, if in a guilty, guilty way, of course I did. That guilt, and the freneticism and fluster of a binge, perhaps detracted from the lingering pleasures of eating as extolled by the Slow Food Movement but, even so, with a binge you are taking in masterful amounts of all the foods you most relish and desire and there is fun and joy to be had in that, is there not? A lot of bulimics and concerned parties who bemoan the binge – the physical consequences and pain and the mental fallout it so cunningly bestows – often forget to mention the upsides. Mainlining on food, for all its shame and shortfalls, does have its ecstatic moments, though perhaps it is not done to admit it. Eventually, though, like so many too-good-for-your-own-good pastimes, they begin to pall. Of course the binge's highs swiftly fail to reach great heights as once they fleetingly did. And its opposite, starvation, the yawning tedium of deprivation, starts to lack lustre and colour after a while; its glamour diminishes and becomes all too drab. So even bulimia's redeeming qualities begin to disappoint and her ugly traits increasingly haunt the mind and linger in all their horror round the body for all to see.

The third reason for giving up on her was perhaps the most tangible. It took the form of Donovan.

After Fred had moved on and until I met Donovan most of the ships I passed were pretty dismal. I suppose I took on that kind of man because I felt they were all I was good for; only if I lost weight could I expect more.

One brief boyfriend never let me meet his friends, the insult of which rankled, though I said nothing, being of the erroneous view that he was better than nothing. One was called Gavin and his notion of romance was to take me to a squat on the Isle of Wight with few windowpanes, no bed and orange thick-pile carpet flattened and encrusted with dubious matter. Another was a handsome ballet dancer called Nigel who was chippy and gay and lived with a vicar in

Hammersmith. I constituted an experiment in bisexuality which was manifestly unsuccessful. Rufus was good and kind, he collected me in his car, walked on the outside of pavements and paid for dinners in smart restaurants, thus displaying a gallantry and generosity that was a novelty to me. (I was used to dates in Pizza Express with men who, when I politely offered to contribute to the bill as my mother had taught me, always said yes and sometimes even made me pay for them too. I never did learn how to be one of those expensive girls who goes through life without ever having to resort to her own wallet.) The problem was that I was a novelty to Rufus. He had had sensational girlfriends in Paris and Milan, spoilt, vulgar and trashy and thin, so though I made him laugh I wasn't the one for him. Mickey the workaholic I met in treatment. He worked in the City and was rich and generous and clever and talked faster than anyone I have ever met. He laughed a lot and very merrily but often had tears in his eyes and was married with a mistress and barking. Another was a sadist who worked in television and nearly killed me on the M1. Something about him gripped my foolish stomach and I lost my appetite and all sense of proportion for six weeks before even I began to see sense and realise that there were aspects to him I found repellent. Another still, a transvestite, I liked and admired and he made me laugh, but I discovered he had a girlfriend and a tendency to complain that my stilettos were not as high as his. Unimaginative of me, I know, but I found that a tad unsettling. And, well, I forget the rest.

Donovan was of a different order.

I met him in a fireplace in Belfast. I was not eating that week and I was cold. The city was freezing in the damp sort of way at which it excels and the flat where I was staying had no heating, only glowing coal in one room into which I pressed myself desperately. I was clinging to my knees in a tight huddle in front of the fire, on the shiny tiles where glowing ash was landing having popped and shot like a star and was fading. He maintains now that I was rude to him then but time has misted his memory and I know he is wrong. One of the curses of feeling overweight most of my life has been that I have almost never had the confidence to be knowingly rude – oh, sometimes how I have longed – or purposefully to piss people off even if beneath my foolish, polite exterior I have had the inclination. When he first came into that room I might, momentarily, have hardly noticed him, my glazed eyes staring longingly into the close, hot orange that was stinging my near-side calf and thigh. I expect when I turned and saw him I was thinking, who is this very young person – he was twenty-one – in his olive-green donkey jacket with lost buttons and wasted Doc Marten boots at the bottom of worn dark jeans, soft Antrim Road voice, butt of a fag in his mouth, showing me photographs he had taken? I was probably wondering if he thought I was fat; for sure I was thinking I was myself, such was my self-absorption, and was he the type likely to judge me on my size and condemn? To be honest, I don't remember much, but I do remember he was gentle and funny and clever and I wasn't rude or intentionally so.

That was February 1992. When I next visited our mutual friends in Belfast they were busy having sex upstairs one afternoon; I was back in the fireplace with a book, and the telephone rang. It was Donovan calling from a pay phone in east Slovakia, where he had been travelling alone for some weeks, and he was in the mood to talk. I spoke English, which was a bonus as he was missing it, and I think I was a familiar and friendly ear. It happened again next visit: hosts again absent above and embroiled, telephone rang, then the soft voice winging its way this time from another distant part of Eastern Europe. Next occasion we met, March 1993, was at a reading in Waterstone's on Charing Cross Road. We were there to support the author from Belfast and his wife, both of whom we loved and who had introduced us. Donovan had joined me in the crowd having arrived a little late, down at heel and long black curls absurd and akimbo, a shambolic and striking figure of just seven stone, eyes bigger than ever in the absence of much flesh surround. He had come straight from Victoria where in the nick he had stepped off a train from Moscow. He had been living there for months on Marlboros and dope and trusty Mars bars. He was gaunt and rather smelly, and a few weeks later I was in Belfast and he joined me on a plane back to London and moved in with me for good, one of the best things that ever happened to me.

That helped.

I would still love you if you were eighteen stone.

That too. I have not ever risked quite that but I like to believe the sentiment is sincerely felt. I have often looked in the mirror and thought I was, might as well have been that weight, like the morning I toppled in front of my helpless father. Now there is a figure beyond, I have said to myself countless times. Those times, however many stone I was, I was going on eighteen.

It is an intimate, scratchy relationship with mirrors that I have; most women do, or so I assume, the ones anything like me. I wonder if they communicate with theirs in the way I do with mine. We have a dialogue, my mirror and I, rather private. Our sallies haven't changed much over the years. Good days and bad.

According to Janet Treasure, Professor of Psychiatry at King's College, London, those with eating disorders either look at themselves in mirrors all the time or avoid them completely. When I had bulimia I was in the first category, checking myself at every opportunity. Sometimes, alone in the flat, I took photographs of myself by the dotted and yellowing glass melded into the front of the antique wardrobe at the end of my bed. I was just in my knickers and bra and the photographs, when developed, would act as reminders, dire warnings to myself not to eat. Once a plumber with a blond moustache and a fat white belly sagging like a beanbag over the waistband of his trousers turned up to mend my boiler, which was attached to the wall in my bedroom. As he groped me, during the unpleasant and shocking process, I watched myself in that mirror – mostly to detach myself from reality, partly to check the roll of my stomach, and I thought thank God mine is not quite as big and ugly as his. In those days I was very dependent on the mirror though the readings I took from it were more often than not upsetting.

Even during those heady, all-too-brief moments when I had lost a bit of weight, the mirror rarely registered the change. Friends told me I was thinner but as I saw myself reflected it seemed I was still burdened with a mass of extraneous flesh. Why this difference of opinion? Couldn't be all down to my friends' politeness, surely. Was my mirror a cast-off from a fairground? But the pillows and books on my bed did not inflate in that same mirror, so why did I?

Nothing wrong with my eyes. What was the mechanism whereby I gained flesh that was, according to others around me, make-believe?

A while ago a Professor at the Department of Clinical Psychology at Liverpool University told me that people with eating disorders see themselves as twenty-five per cent fatter than they actually are, and 'normal' women fifteen per cent. This perception of increased girth, he said, is one of the most complex disorders there is. He cited a study that had found a significant correlation between resting metabolic rates in relation to emotional judgements of body size. The biological effect of a reduced metabolic rate can lead to feelings of sluggishness which in turn can be misinterpreted as feelings of being fat.

Janet Treasure told me the image on the retina is fine but the nervous connections can be interfered with, which causes it to be exaggerated along the way. After eating a cake, she says, a woman may think she can actually see her bottom sprouting. The vivid imagery is related to fears and worries, specifically about becoming fat. There is a line between this imagery and hallucination but they are on the same spectrum.

I had heard that emotions can affect how people appraise themselves cognitively; it is obvious I suppose and am sure it is true, it is just hard to accept. These days, now that I am normal-abnormal, I look in my mirror and try to imagine the image that I see before me with fifteen per cent less fat on it and endeavour to believe that that is nearer the true me, but I usually fail. More often than not I take the image as read.

Although when we overeat and then look in the mirror we can, as Treasure says, see our bottoms sprouting (or, in the past in my case, the fast-forward development of another stomach roll, the stomach being the main focus of my narrative), we know in our heart of hearts that it is an illusion and not really to be relied upon. One of the great cruelties of weight loss and gain, it seems to me, is the actual real-time lag between cause and effect. As I eat something, in Salman Rushdie's famous words, naughty but nice, I often wish that its fat-giving properties would immediately and truthfully show themselves for what they are, instantly reflect themselves back to me all the better to stop me from carrying on. A moment on the lips, a lifetime on the hips, or so the pious saying goes. How long does it actually take the ice cream, having hit the lips, to reach its resting place? And though its resting place might feel like the hips or stomach, even look like it to eyes with which emotion has tampered, where does it actually end up?

The time of digestion is three hours or so. Then the deconstructed calories exist as a resource which can be called upon for energy. As Treasure says, it depends where they go. They can instantly get the call-up and be burned off with exercise, or be laid down as fat-in-waiting temporarily or for ever. Professor Bloom told me that when you gain weight the number of fat cells do not increase but the existing ones each store more fat. They take on 'fatty acids' from the blood-stream (which arrive there from food) and so if you eat unsaturated fat, which is rather liquid, you too become rather flabby.

'Which fat cells store the most fat,' Bloom says, 'is age and sex dependent, but how we don't understand. Thus girls have more fat underneath the skin all over (which makes for rounded contours), but especially around the hips, buttocks and breasts. The latter specialised distribution becomes more marked with age, while the general underskin fat becomes

177

less, giving rise to haggard looks with a big bum. With men, fat redistributes to the centre of the body, particularly inside the (pot) belly with age. Both men and women take less exercise and eat more food as they age so they gain weight in general.'

There have been a few mirrors in my life, some more supportive than others. I'll never forget a speaking glass, not strictly a mirror, that I lingered in front of once in my twenties in a street in Paris; only in Paris. It was a patisserie shop window. The cakes inside were like ballerinas, light and flouncy and all the colours you would see in a Christmas production of *The Nutcracker*. Little mauve mousselines aglaze with blackcurrants; small pastries filled with crème anglaise and raspberries or topped with shavings of white, milk and dark chocolate done up like theatrical hairdos; delicate croissants with almonds and icing sugar and more and more besides. I looked at them a while, in their endless rows as orderly and disciplined as a corps de ballet, hungry and tempted but not quite giving in. And as I was grappling with myself, voices in my head both urging me to enter the shop and begging me not to, I heard another voice, a male one, behind me. '*Attention kilos!*' it cackled, and as it did so my own reflection moved into focus at the forefront of the window's vast viewfinder and seemed fit to fill the very surface of the substantial glass and to enlarge before my eyes. It was the thought of giving into these beautiful, magical, disturbing fancies. The window's close-up malice had room only for me and none left for the speaker. I turned quickly to see him, a man in his forties, neat and chic and rich and smug with clicking heels beneath expensive shoes, couture coat and jaunty hat disappearing from view, carrying with him his briefcase and his disapprobation. I took a deep breath and immediately ran in the other direction, never to return.

Not all looking glasses are so malign but even as a rare shopper I can say with certainty that some shops have fortunate mirrors in their changing rooms and others have ones that are hideous. Those at Marks and Spencer, marred with lighting as would befit a morgue, give rise to deathly shapes and hues. In them my thighs and bum look the same colour and texture as cauliflowers and I both believe and don't believe them. I know they are telling the truth, but a truth for that instant alone and for my eyes only. I console myself with the thought that no one else will ever see me thus, naked beneath neon, with the possible exception of my undertaker, and in his company, who knows, I might be past caring. For the time being that truth can remain hidden under my dark clothes and the gentler light of London days and lamps with bulbs of yolkier watts.

In some shops, on the other hand, they have vast mirrors which lean elegantly backwards and are graced with intelligent lighting. I don't know if these have had dubious things done to their mirrors to lull customers into a false sense of security and spending, but many men and women certainly step out of them feeling lighter of both kinds of pounds. Of course when we get home and try on the new skirt in front of our own mirrors things never seem quite as rosy. Then I tell myself to try to retain the original image, an image in the shop which had its place, and might again still in some kind person's eyes, in some sombrely lit place, somewhere, sometime.

I know really that you can't trust shop mirrors. I think most women know, deep down, that they are never quite as sincere as those at home. We are aware that with them the marketing men have had some kind of truck so as to make us look better than we really do. It cannot just be the lighting. Is it something genius in the angle? Friends say it is a clever bending and they're probably right, but I can't quite understand how it works so on the whole choose to overlook the fact and continue to fall for the ploy.

Mirrors at home are more honest. Their provenance is likely to have been a Homebase or high-street bathroom shop more intent on selling scalloped sanitary ware, I think they call it, than making our bodies acceptable in clothes. There is a mirror in my mother and stepfather's bathroom which has been there for twenty-five years and is brutal. It never fails to upset me and pitch me into a gloom and I never look in it unless I stray past and by mistake happen to glance. In another bathroom along the corridor is another full-length number, infinitely more sympathetic, actively kind I would say, which I always visit and which never fails to deliver a momentary lift. Neither of these mirrors is specialised, one pinned to the inside of a cupboard, the other with its original sales sticker scruffily still half-stuck to it, hanging on to a papery wall. No clever lighting within range. I wonder how much their respective characters are my imagination. Certainly my mother has never mentioned that hers is a bully. She wafts to and fro, sometimes almost tap dances in front of it in her vintage clothes and paste jewels, and they seem to get on just fine, their relationship is sweet. I suspect I formed my entrenched opinion about these two mirrors years ago. Perhaps I once looked at the 'kind' one at the start of a Not Especially Fat day and at the 'cruel' one at the end of it, following a twelve-hour period, all too common at my mother's, of overeating, breakfast, lunch, tea and dinner and picking in between, and I embraced some conclusions based wholly on the fallout of emotions.

Breakfast, whenever I went back to my mother's house for a weekend, used unwelcomely to hove into view. The kitchen would be full of sun and papers and the smell of croissants and toast. There I could not help it, I would become a breakfasting non-breakfaster giving in to breakfast. By the time I had also scoffed a big lunch, well, all was lost for the day so I might as well really go for it and have *tea* too. Tea was always the troublesome one. It tested me more than most because it was such a novelty and so utterly irresistible.

The kitchen in Oxford is a beautiful yellow, nothing as sour as lemon or crude orange as egg yolk but rich and warm as sunlight. There is a large table with a dog-eared sofa at one end and a variety of old mugs hanging on hooks in the alcove. There are three paintings in oil so thick you could pick the strokes off the canvases like scabs. They are of Brighton Pier, a figure beneath an umbrella and a silhouetted couple behind a windbreaker on a beach. Their colours are so bright people are struck by them as they enter the room for the first time, and even in winter, with the curtains closed by tea-time and the lights soft, they are more subdued and cosy but still startle. My mother puts a cluster of mugs on the faded Indian cotton tablecloth, a pile of knives and plates. The china is all different, odd bits that have survived the years, but my favourite is white with two thick stripes round the rim in turquoise and yellow. On the side there are packets of muffins and crumpets and outsize loaves for those who prefer toast. Butter in a pottery dish, olive oil spread for my stepfather who watches his cholesterol. There is a dented tin with coffee and walnut cake or heavy home-made ginger cake, or chocolate brownies. Tea itself is in a squat silver pot that belonged to my father's family and looks as if it would only need a gentle shine to conjure up a genie. It is dented and leaky and its inside blackened by years of Earl Grey and lapsang, but it retains a battered elegance and tea-time would not be the same without it.

I think of tea – by which I mean scones and biscuits and cucumber sandwiches and cakes and not the proper meal also known as high tea – as a generational thing. My generation, while they may nab a cup of tea around five-ish and possibly an energy bar if they feel a bit peckish, do not go in for any such old-fashioned malarkey. Modern life would seem to preclude the time to make real cakes every day or people carefree enough to eat them regularly. Outside the homes of the under-fifties, tea only ever properly takes place in nursing homes or grand hotels where special patisserie chefs daily prepare fondant fancies. They are displayed on four-storey plates and passed round foyers overwrought with palms and pianos which have no feeling of the real world, and they are eaten by the type of hushed folk who appear to live at a different pace from the rest of us. Certainly tea is a meal my contemporaries have for the most part shelved, except maybe on the odd weekend in the country or when visiting an aged aunt. In my mind at least it remains something I associate pretty well entirely with Oxford and the past.

When we moved to Oxford and my oldest best friend Miranda came to the university, I used to ask her and several other hungry undergraduates to visit. They often dropped by around tea-time and seemed grateful for a proper fire and stacks of free crumpets engorged with melting butter.

These days weekend tea-time in Oxford hails a break in the

afternoon's cold outdoor activities with the children, the moment to reward their expended energy with pasta, sausages and broccoli, apples, yoghurts and brownies, and ours with muffins and gingernuts. Sometimes Mum and James invite their friends to come and join in and it is a chaotic occasion of adult conversation trying to prevail above cries for ketchup and cake. A few years ago I made a rule to myself that breakfast and tea at Oxford were off limits but it is a rule I have been known to break. Odd times the ends of my sons' sausages or a discarded slice of toasted malt loaf just cannot be thrown away and it is me upon whom they are not wasted. Before I had children of my own I remember mothers bemoaning the fact that picking at the leftovers of their children's tea was their undoing. I wondered then what could have been so tempting about a forkful of nibbled chicken nugget and noodle made cold by HP sauce and rejection, but now I know. By tea-time, the blood sugar quite spent in the face of all-boyish pursuits, punches and pistols, I can see the merits in even the most lumpen gob of Bolognese or a bonsai of broccoli at its most forlorn. At home the picking is contained, just enough to give me the little lift necessary in the run-up to the boys' bath-time. But in the persuasive atmosphere of the Oxford kitchen at tea-time, one mouthful of fish finger leads to another and then in a funny way to a biscuit here and slice of cake there, and before you know it upstairs your stomach is not fit for surveillance, even in the more soothing mirror of the two, but those mouthfuls were so delicious they were worth it and after a fashion you don't really care.

My current mirrors at home include a hand mirror with normal glass on one side and the magnifying type on the other, but I don't really count that one. It is good for pointing up blemishes on the face and for enabling me to apply mascara not too messily, but it can never take in the whole of me. Two mirrors in the bathroom are bigger but not much better. One only ever watches me brushing my teeth and cuts me off at the waist, no bad thing but hardly realistic. The other, an old one, colour of raw egg white and with speckles, when I'm standing up in the bath only captures my middle. In fact, it can be quite thoughtful to my middle but only because my middle, lacking chest and head and calves and feet, is out of context. Pieced back together in a long mirror it never looks so well. I think of that elderly mirror as kind but not very sincere. My main mirror, modern, bog-standard, plain, full-length, hangs on the inside of the cupboard in our bedroom. When I open the door to look at myself once maybe twice a day, the hinges squeak and I tense a little every time. There is a feeble light inside the cupboard. Even during the day I am never seeing myself in raw light that would give the real picture, but mostly that suits and deludes me just fine.

Sometimes I look in the mirror in my clothes, sometimes not. Looking at my body unadorned is a particular challenge because its imperfections are so barefaced.

Clothed or unclothed, I strike poses. Clothed or unclothed, some make me look fatter than others. Good ones enable me to close the cupboard door, go downstairs and face the world if not with confidence then at least with benign resignation. Bad ones constitute a sport of sorts, a challenge to the strength of that day's psyche.

I find if I stand sideways, put my hand on my hip, elbow sticking out at a studiously carefree angle, and take a sharp intake of breath as a means of disciplining my stomach, the effect is not altogether disastrous. Sometimes my arm stretched backwards in that rather exaggerated way can seem quite lean, but never as lean as my sinewy friend's. Her arms have a tell-tale vein running down them that only really thin people ever have. God knows where my arm vein went. Sometimes wonder if I've even got one. The curve of my stomach can seem shallower when I lift my ribs and strike my bum out backwards in a particular way, though not too far else the bum itself enlarges. Get it spot on and I can find myself feeling only a few degrees off pleased. If I stand straight-on, keeping one leg bent and outwards just so, I can usually stave off immediate decline. Alarming is when I stand with my back to the mirror and turn my head, only to see a hippo-bottom filling the whole surface of the glass, or stand full-on, leaning slightly backwards, which does untold damage to the thighs. They expand before my eyes into calumphing triangular bags of flesh with what look like moulded pockets at each side in which I keep slabs of lard. It is mild masochism that dares me to try these unfortunate poses at all and I am not sure really why I do it. I guess if a positive pose has given rise to a glimmer of hope, then a negative one injects a little balance. I never want to delude myself that I look more than passable, let alone good. Better to be one's own fiercest critic lest complacency should ever overtake self-doubt.

I never spend very long in front of the mirror. It is quick assessments I go in for because it only takes a minute or two to get the picture and there is not much I can do immediately to change things. I mean, the poses are all well and dandy for the mirror but it is faintly pointless perfecting them for hours on end only to abandon them the moment one steps away from it. I am not dedicated or interested enough to remember later to stand or sit in the ways that showed me to better advantage or to avoid those which manifestly did not. I expect there are women who are practised in the art of standing 'correctly' so their legs look longer and stomachs flatter or whatever, but not the kind of women I have ever met. I find in real life I have to exist as a human being, not a statue, and anyway don't have the time or the head for it. I have to crawl bum in the air under the kitchen table with a dustpan and brush; I have to form my hip into a bungy seat for the baby; I ungainly run down the street in a hurry while clutching my coat against the cold. I have to lollop with heavy bags from Tesco; gather together my son's football kit in time; balance on a stool at (the end of) a (shady) bar; slouch in front of the telly with a chocolate. I have to walk and move and rush and talk and eat and try to get comfortable and forget how I look for hours at a time as I interview a man about his job analysing snot samples at Hammersmith Hospital; have conversations about nits and reading books and tantrums with other parents at the school gate; play dinosaurs and tiger cubs with my children on the floor and encourage them to learn how to spell broccoli and because; talk to a builder about desludging the radiators; grab a movie and pizza and a precious word with my husband away from little boys. If I was busy trying to stick to my better poses whenever I was in company, I would not be able to listen or speak for the concentration of it. I would have to turn myself into a foolish statue, and I would look not only still too fat for my liking but off my rocker besides.

So I suppose the brief posing must be done for confirmation that one is a fat and ugly old goat or, more, in the hope of a momentary modicum of reassurance that one is not. I think my relationship with the mirror is fairly pointless as it invariably sees me as others do not, and I am not really looking into it to know what *it* thinks but to imagine what others might, something upon which it can never shed light. I know this because I occasionally watch other women in mirrors, twitching at a piece of hair, meddling with a skirt, doing little steps and turns this way and that, almost dances. Their eyes reveal that they are thinking a thousand things, that their brain is going click click click like a taxi meter with extravagant figures and calculations, and I know that not one of their thoughts is anything like what anyone else within a few yards of them is thinking. We look at others in mirrors (and in life) with envy or indifference. We look at ourselves in mirrors inaccurately and all too often with disbelief mixed unfairly and squarely with a familiar dose of dismay.

I do understand why some women dispense with them entirely, it can be quite an effective form of forgetting though never entirely so. No one can overlook their body altogether. Every time you pull off a jersey you are confronted by arms and breasts; every time you do up the zip of a skirt there is a bright wobble of hip with which you must negotiate; every time you sit down there is your stomach hoving into view and there are your thighs spreading across the chair with an enthusiasm you cannot fail to notice and resent. And avoiding mirrors completely must constitute an art in itself. I wonder at the person who never catches herself in the windscreen mirror or the surround mirrors in the loos at a cinema or motorway service station. She must be very alert. Even when I do not want to see myself on Very Fat days, I am constantly wrong-footed by unplanned glances. They come at me like hiccups, unexpected, unwelcome but unavoidable, and I am usually forced to give in to them and try to think, what the hell.

Those who never look in mirrors may lay claims to disinterest or lack of time, but the real reason has got to be more to do with hating the way they look, does it not? To be honest, when I'm on a mission to avoid myself that is my reason. Most women feel too fat and have bits of their body they would like to lop off and have some moments or days when they can't face a mirror, but the majority of us do not hate ourselves so much that we do not wish to confront ourselves at all. Sometimes, on a Very Fat day and when I have a serious case of clarty, I might find I am in too much of a hurry to face myself in my cupboard and rush away and out without the usual check-up. On the whole though, my meeting with the mirror is as routine as that with my toothbrush, if a bit more loaded. Used in conjunction with my scales it has some bearing on my mood for the day and the decisions about what I am and am not allowed to wear and eat, but not completely. More often than not I forget its instructions to me the moment I have left its side and embarked on the rest of my day. Give or take the usual fifteen per cent here or there, our partnership is healthy enough, I suppose. If you have regular encounters with mirrors, feelings of dismay are as likely as not but those of complete surprise can almost never be.

Dinner

I think when Donovan moved in it was all over quite quickly.

After a few weeks we went to the wedding in New York of a couple of friends and I don't remember bulimia making the trip. That I made the wedding at all is testimony to that fact. It was the first big social occasion I had managed to attend in quite a while, or certainly the first for years I remember with any degree of pleasure. There were a number of celebration lunches and dinners with a gang of close friends over several days and I joined in them all with gusto and little concern for my troublesome stomach as far as I recall. The pair of us carried on our journey to Mexico in a challenging Greyhound bus, stopping off in New Orleans for magnificent Caesar salads and, once across the border, for gooey enchiladas produced from wooden huts. Even I spurned one filled with mince and chilli and melted cheese and covered in chocolate sauce, not for considerations of weight but just because that was a combination, call me old-fashioned, that on the whole I'd really rather not. (My father, crossing the Empty Quarter in 1967, happily went with the flow and ate sheeps' eyeballs and bollocks. Alas, I did not inherit his spirit of adventure.) And in the fishing village of San Blas I was more concerned that I was being eaten alive by mosquitos (I landed seventy-two bites in a couple of hours) than with the wearisome business of eating myself.

Back at home, in our early days, we used to go out to eat quite often, to various cafés and pizza places, so as not always to have to prepare food ourselves. It unsettled me still, the messy and unpredictable nature of cooking in a flat with a kitchen the size of a piece of A4, the messy and unpredictable nature of cooking full stop, and tricky associations following years of Lean Cuisine, Slimfast and solitary control. I am not a good or natural cook. I can make about a dozen things well enough and still like to look at sumptuous photographs of food in our fat cookery books but rarely do I push the boat out enough actually to attempt the recipes they illustrate. I read them avidly and fill myself with good and bad intentions never fulfilled. The looking gives me pleasure but the doing can occasionally be a frightening prospect – the potential for overeating, the chaos in the kitchen, the unknown.

My aunt Trish always told me I would never get a husband if I did not start to cook. She is of the school that believes the way to a man's heart is through his stomach. 'It's regrettable but true,' she often said. Fortunately Donovan, very much a baguette, cheese and salami type, was tolerant and did not seem to mind that I wasn't rustling up impossible poussins and squid ink soufflés. He likes to cook and eat but back then was too diverted by photography and his mixtures more chemical than edible – he spent more time in our tiny bathroom (which since his addition in my life had swiftly been converted into a darkroom) than at the stove. Once he was making curry that called for a pinch of a particular spice and asked, 'How much is a pinch?' Another time he did attempt a tomato risotto from a mumsy book which was so disgusting we both snorted with derision and promptly dialled up a local pizza.

His work took him away a great deal: one nine-week trip at one point, and a couple of others for a good six, were just a few among many – for me at any rate – longueurs. Even during those stints when I missed him massively and might have seized the opportunity to diet and stray back into old habits, I ate as 'normally' as I had ever done before contracting an eating disorder, if with new-found care. I created systems that involved a certain amount of sensible compensation – if I had given in to a pudding the night before, I might cut the bread at lunch the next day and just opt for salad – but nothing like the bulimia-scale compensation of starvation to offset a binge.

He said he liked me as I was, that proportion in a woman was what was pleasing in his book not size itself, and he encouraged chocolates and the rest because he knew they made me happy. He wasn't worried about their consequences and felt that nor should I be. It did all slowly drip-drip into my consciousness but the difficulty was that the worry was so long-term ingrained that while I could keep it in check, I was never able to slough it off entirely. With the arrival in my life of a partner who sincerely did not notice if I gained or shed a few pounds and certainly did not appear to care, I set to wondering, as I persisted with my normal-abnormal low-key anxiety, who on earth my quest to be thin was precisely *for* any more?

In the past the answer might have been men, possibly starting with my father.

Approbation from my father was so much less easily won than from my mother. Hers flowed readily and almost without my having to make any effort. He was always a harder nut to crack. I spent my childhood and youth desperately seeking to acquire his rare compliments and shots of approval. What with an empty head that he had led me to believe was probably terminal, I had the impression that the simplest route to acceptance was by gaining if not a mind then at least a figure that he could admire.

I do not think I could have been more wrong. Although he called me greedy when I was very young, I now feel sure, and have for a while in the light of adulthood and perspective, that they were just draughty remarks he was making. They were more likely spoken in the spirit of passing irritation, teasing or affection than fundamental criticism. I recognised long before I met Donovan that Pop was far more concerned about my brain than my looks. It was not that he thought looks did not matter – he appreciated beauty and would have been worried had I become obese – more that it was my brain that needed fixing. He felt my body, though it tended to a plumpness which required the occasional pointing out, was not alarming. After the age of about fourteen he did not remark upon my greed or size and the notion that he cared a great deal was entirely a whim of my imagination, bred of reading too much into the word greedy. The truth, which began to dawn on me as I passed through my twenties, was that he loved me to share and appreciate the pleasures of delicious food with him and only wished for me to be happy, regardless of my size. (Quite often I would ask him if he had any ideas about what I should be in life and he would exasperate me by answering unhelpfully that he did not mind, he cared only that I should be happy and should not be an actress.) Whenever he came to London he never failed to take me and my half-brothers and -sisters to a

French restaurant in which he had an interest. There he encouraged us to try sweetbreads and snails, pigs' trotters and langoustines, and sincerely urged upon me crème brûlées and the signature plate of different sorbets made from mangoes and kiwis and passionfruits and blackcurrants.

The year that Donovan moved in with me, Pop left France and returned to England for good. For ten years, from nineteen to twenty-nine, I had used up a large proportion of my earnings by visiting him two or three times a year, every holiday I had. No question I wanted to be there with him and he was always very keen for me to go, but we had our ups and downs. One time we clashed to such an extent that I told him I had had enough and was leaving. He apologised and begged me to stay. I refused and bagged a lift back to London with a friend, cursing him all the way. Another time I was in a bad car crash on a winding road above a gorge. I broke my sternum and could not move for the pain. He came to the hospital with baguettes and *brandade de morue* (a pâté made with salt cod and olive oil) and cheeses from the goats on the hill and made me laugh so much we could hear the bone clicking in my breast. Other times he welcomed my friends to stay and took us on expeditions to beautiful towns and villages and markets and restaurants and dinners with his local friends. One year I proposed that Hugh, a friend of mine who was between jobs and broke, should come and look after him. He was funny and a brilliant cook, so Pop felt a particular gratitude to me for that suggestion. Between shifts working at his computer, Pop would earnestly discuss recipes with Hugh and they trawled the markets together and came up with simple but perfect dinners of creamy spinach with mussels and lemon and almond tarts, which I was always urged at length to review.

Pop moved to an apartment in a haunted tweed mill in

Oxfordshire. His beautiful pictures hung on the exposed brick walls beneath the rust-red, industrial metal beams. He zipped about the pale wooden floor in his nippy electric 'Squirrel' wheelchair, but for all his evident pleasure to be closer to family and old friends he was becoming progressively more unwell. He needed two full-time helpers because the stiffness, pains and ailments caused by long-term muscular dystrophy and mishaps – he had been blown up by a land mine in the Sahara, had a ludicrous number of car crashes over the years, had suffered crushed vertebrae in India and broken legs in France – were such that no one person could lift him. He had a breathing machine at night and in order to sleep he would have to be turned several times by skilful hands that would not hurt him. My six-pack brother Nat took months off to look after him full-time; my sister Sabrina and her son travelled from America; and Pop's brother, ex-sister-in-law and three ex-wives (plus some of their later husbands) visited him as frequently as geography would allow. My mother, being only forty minutes away, went to see him three times a week bearing baskets of books, snowdrops and marmalades as well as an enduring willingness to help him sort out his financial perils. He gave her short-shrift sometimes, some of his erstwhile cruelty coming out, but he depended on and trusted her, enjoyed her company, and she forgave him everything. My stepfather James and their daughter/my half-sister, Eugenie, sometimes went along with her. Donovan and I stayed for weekends. Because my father's time was evidently if gradually running out, and because I was older and so a jot less empty of head, and happier, there were no more of the ups and the downs. We gossiped and giggled and Pop always took enormous trouble to produce impressive lunches and dinners, either at the hands of my brother Nat with his chefly skills or by coaxing the best from the kindly but less culinary young men who also cared for him. Pop, his appetite reduced by nauseous drugs and the indignity he had always dreaded of needing someone else to cut up his food, ate like a sparrow but he continued to insist that everyone else, including myself, should gobble up with gusto.

It may have once been for my father I was trying to be thin, but not since my early twenties.

So if not for him, then was it for other men? The obvious answer that I might have wanted to be thin for men in general sticks in my gullet. But I reluctantly admit, though rather a damning indictment of my character, that before I met Donovan I half-believed if I remained fat I would never be attractive to a member of the opposite sex or, if I was, certainly not for long enough to sustain a lasting association.

I say half-believed because when Fred painted my picture again and again and when the Scottish novelist forgot to be derogatory about my stomach, I did recognise there were a few men for whom skin and bones did not mean a whole heap. There again, maybe they were just being polite, albeit politeness which they managed to sustain day and night for the years (in Fred's case) or months (in Hugo's) that I was with them and the subsequent decades across which we have remained friends. I could not quite square that at the time, though when those relationships foundered I did wonder if their overlooking my size might not have been politeness all along. I thought things were over because, even though couched differently and more kindly, bottom line these men no longer found me attractive. My friends, all of whom I considered to be thinner than me, were in long-term relationships or married, so on some level I must have surmised that I was too fat. The subsequent passing ships did little to detract from this view. They were all invariably wrecked 'ere long but only ever upon that fatal obstacle that was my iceberg stomach, never upon such dangers as the rocks of mutual disinterest or the storms of mismatched personalities.

Donovan and I had a monumental falling out in a shopping centre. We were going at a different pace; no specific obstacles, just I was on miles per hour and he was on knots. We split up in the Marks and Spencer food hall next to the thick and creamy custard, and my stomach contracted tightly like a flouncy sea creature under attack from an enemy. The next morning he woke me around four and invited me to go on a walk with him. Three months later we were married.

I do not think I am being controversial if I say that women who go in for weddings usually go in for diets during the lead-up to their big day. Losing weight is there on the checklist along with all the other crucial business such as booking the vicar, sending out the invitations, calling the caterers and choosing the dress. Many succeed because it is the one occasion perhaps in their whole life, more so than any birthday or graduation ceremony or other rite of passage, when they are going to be on show for all the people they most care about (and some they do not) to see and appraise them. If you can't manage to shed some excess and be beautiful on your wedding day – and as we all know, hey-ho, beauty is thin, thin is beauty – then whenever can you? Women married a while show you their wedding photographs and it is no coincidence that many do so with a sigh and the wistful words, 'Look how thin I was!' I was aware of the pressure. 'What's the dress going to be like?' asked friends and strangers alike on learning that I had become engaged, and, 'How much are you hoping to lose? How many weeks you got?' I knew I ought to diet; it is part of the ritual. But, curiously, I was not feeling particularly fat and never quite got round to it.

I wore a simple dress made of soft, plain, duchesse satin which seemed both to flow and nearly crunch like dry grass as I moved. The colour was ivory or parchment or oyster or champagne, or whatever fancy name people call cream when referring to wedding dresses. Mum designed it. Narrow waist, slight bustle at the back, tight sleeves reaching in a point over knuckles which a couple of decades earlier had at last lost their dimples and discovered bones. She found a short length of antique braid made with seed pearls to go across the low, Tudor-esque neckline and a frail veil of old lace. Looking back at the pictures I can just see the inside of the church with its tremulous candles on every window ledge and the arch over the aisle of silver birch trees, fairy lights attached to their bare branches. I can once again immediately conjure up the cold, smell the incense and hear Elgar's *Nimrod* and the drag and swish of the bouquet held not in front of me but downwards, ivy-trailing beside my father and I along the aisle, and the vows. I can see the vast fire in the warm, dark dining hall of the small Oxford college where we had the reception, almost taste the food arranged by my father and made by the excellent college chef: the scallop and bacon salad, the *pollo surpriso* for nostalgia's sake, the dotted vanilla ice cream and French chocolate mousse cake. Can see the generous expressions of ninety close family and friends and Donovan beside me all the while with his black velvet suit with its black velvet buttons and purple silk tie and his tight hand. I feel my smile which made my muscles ache but which I could not stop and can detect a slight sling of stomach and can see a way to it, it has a certain something. It is a part of me.

Men love their wives or partners or they do not, obviously, and our weight, the amount I am talking about at any rate, is not going to make them love us more or less. Most men, if pressed, and I go in for pressing, say that within 'normal' parameters – which, think Donovan's eighteen stone, are heaps wider than women's – they do not mind about their partner's size. Even if it might have had some bearing once, along with all the other factors which constitute a first impression, it is not what is interesting about a person. A lot of the men I respect don't think about or notice it much (the ones who do I find rather suspect), unless their partner becomes fat or thin to a dangerous degree (in which case fair do's as it is then a health concern). Certainly, many just want the normal-abnormal women they are with to be rid of this preoccupation with weight, this mild lunacy (I speak for myself), to forget about it once and for all. It is tedious and unsexy. I do know this, as I know that thin people fall in and out of love just as much as fatter ones do. Being thin is no insurance. If it was, only fat people would ever get divorced. This equation is risibly simplistic but needs to be drummed into people like me because there remains a stupid part of us – me – that thinks being thin means getting to be loved in the first place and then being enduringly loveable. I think just a few pounds off – perhaps? After all most men, even if like Donovan they say they don't, surely take a view; they must do, mustn't they, deep-down?

I do have one or two friends whose partners tell them to go on diets. That is territory into which mine would never stray. I have him better trained. He once told me that if I was worried about my weight maybe, for my own sake, not his, I should do a little exercise. I practically unravelled and he has never been allowed to forget it. My friend Laura says it is a tightrope of tact her husband must tread. Often she asks if something makes her look fat. If he says, maybe, a little bit, round the bum/hips/tummy, she feels upset and angry. There again, for him to tell her the dress/trousers or whatever looks lovely on her is to invite accusations that he is a liar. She says he cannot get it right because, 'poor love, there is no right!'

I once overheard a man in a café say to his wife, whom I know vaguely, 'No chocolate torte for you, my darling, remember your stomach! Ha! ha!' Ha ha, I nearly fell off my chair. This husband is squat and portly with a hammock for a double chin besides. This wife is a woman who has been denying herself on and off all her life. It is not as if she isn't critical enough of herself already without his input. She eats like a rabbit, just lettuce and carrots most of the time with sudden bursts of quantities of chocolate and chips in between. I believe she is beautiful but, married to him, she believes her bum is destined to be fat and to become fatter for all eternity.

Some women are obeying orders from a particular man. They are fighting to remain attractive to a person for whom their weight is a big deal. In many cases, like mine, our partners are not imposing the struggle upon us; we are imposing it upon ourselves. We kid ourselves that the way to remain attractive to them is by being thin, even though these very men have told us umpteen times they don't necessarily find thin attractive and insist they would still love us any which way.

Perhaps it is not about one man, then, but about men in general?

At times in my life, when the irrational became too over-bearing, I think I thought that if I were thin I would attract lots and lots of men. I should like to be able to credit myself with more intelligence, but my logic lacking much reason did go something along those lines. Perhaps the thinking was that if I were thin I would attract the optimum number of men for an optimum amount of time, that that was Thin's holy grail. With what in mind, I am not quite sure. Whether I planned, as this mythical thin person, to sleep with all these mythical men that my thinness was bound to send into a lustful spin, I am not entirely sure. It has to be said that the crude prize of quantity I managed to pull off without being thin and I knew it was a waste of time; more than a waste of time, it was frequently excruciating. So perhaps wanting to be thin so as to have men gasping, or so I liked to picture it, was about achieving that fashionable notion, choice. If I was thin I could unceremoniously see off the unsuitable passing ships which fat women often feel are their due and with which they make do for fear nothing better will materialise. I could make my way without passing Go directly to men who were more appreciative and worthwhile and steadfast and loving! Geronimo.

Trouble was, I never did become thin enough for long enough to find out. And even as a theory it was flawed. First, I knew attraction inspired by physical appearance alone was superficial and therefore not desirable. Second, while I remained fat(ish) I came across anomalies who seemed happy for me not to alter the status quo. Most notably Donovan, who says the right things, has stuck by me through fat and thin and who married me for God's sake, so appears actually to mean them. Donovan, who has single-handedly turned my topsy-turvy beliefs on their heads. I do still – partly – abide by these skewed beliefs and even now, in my current circumstances, fantasise once in a while about this me that is mythically thin. But at least these days, progress of sorts, I am interrogating myself with the question, why on earth?

Why on earth?

Still to prompt in all these mythical men a lustful spin? I mean, what in heaven's name would be the point? For the sake of potential sex with mythical men with whom I don't want sex? All those chocolates across all these years denied for *that*? For the sport of watching men attracted then rejected? In which case it is about power and not sex at all, and surely there are easier ways – if power is your bag though it is not mine – of being powerful without pretending for ever that you hate chocolate or being on a permanent diet?

No, if it was about and for men once it is not now.

The people for whom we want to be thin, or so we tell ourselves and are so often given to believe, are not men but other women.

I have thought about this one long and hard and know that it carries some weight, but only up to a point because it does beg the question, which women?

If you try to pin them down you discover they elude you. Which women? Strangers we pass in the street, salesgirls in shops? All that gruesomely dull dieting and heartbreak over lost breakfasts just on the off chance that a fleeting woman might be prompted to think, 'She's thin,' and even if she did we would never know. Couldn't be. Then for other women at work or at social gatherings and parties, acquaintances merely, even those in familiar settings whom we don't know but might just be introduced to? Is all that dedication to the scales and head destruction really worth the effort for the reward of a once-over by someone we half-know and if we got to know better may not even like?

Women family members, then, and friends; those we know and love and care about, and the ones who care about us? We do it for them, I wonder. But which ones *exactly* and why?

My mother?

Today she uttered to me the immortal line, 'Here, have some of this celery, it is delicious.' Celery is a pleasing green, it has attributes of length and crunchiness, I own, but one thing it can never naked be is delicious. The view that celery is delicious is that of someone who in her system has clocked that it famously contains fewer calories than are used to chew it up and marked it with a large tick; someone who has contemplated for a fair few years the subject of denial and minds about staying trim. My mother has high standards. Perhaps it is for her I want to be thin. I wish to make her happy and proud.

But this is not really logical. Of all the people in all the world, she is the one on whom I really can rely to love me whatever my size, the unconditional nature of maternal love and all that. (Donovan's generous leeway of eighteen stone, though I've no intentions of finding out, may just crack under the strain of nineteen.) And anyway, there are easier and better ways to prompt in her feelings of happiness and pride than being thin, like never forgetting to write thank-you letters, like making her laugh, like producing bouncing grandchildren. Losing weight is more complex and less efficient. If ever I become marginally thinner than my norm she spots it a mile off and comments. She is pleased after a fashion but she also worries in a way that only mothers do and says my face looks older and more gaunt and my wrist bones are like a sparrow's (my father always said she did a good line in exaggeration) and I should be careful of osteoporosis and here I brought you some steak and cake.

No, while I might have copied some of her ways and inherited from her a few ideas and beliefs regarding the benefits of a light lunch and a small waist, I know that she does not really mind. I like to think her comments about people's size and physical appearance are due to a keener sense of the detail of the world around her than most. Mum has synaesthesia, her senses singularly heightened, vision with sound. It means that, for her, hearing various words produces a particular colour in her mind's eye: Monday is pink, Thursday blue. Certain shapes and colours give her real joy or cause real offence. She has to avert her eyes from such chemically mixed insults as Barclays Bank turquoise. It is a condition which means she looks and observes and sees and cares in ways which most of us do not. She can walk into a derelict house and an image of how it could be, after the builders and decorators have done her bidding, superimposes itself on the reality before her. It is a visual talent which passed me by. Landscapes, buildings, people, in all their peculiar and infinite variety, their beauty and ugliness, rivet her, and size comes into that. She owns up to an interest in how people look. Some of it must be to do with the superficial aesthetic of thinness imposed by a culture obsessed and to which we all attend, but with her it is also about an aesthetic which is all her own. She appreciates a delicate ankle or long limb with a painterly eye but her driving ambition as a mother is that her daughters be happy, fulfilled at work and married, not thin. I am not wanting to be thin on her account. There are many aspects of life about which I request and value her opinion and wisdom and humour but weight is not one of them. In fact I feel a kind of adolescent irritation if she comments on any aspect of my physical appearance or size. Sometimes she tells me my hair could do with a bit of conditioner or a brush. Sometimes she tells me that a skirt looks nice on me. Sometimes if I wear a spot of uncharacteristic red (only ever a scarf at most and then only ever at Christmas) she expresses disproportionate delight and joy at the relief from my relentless black. Sometimes she tells me she cannot understand why I have given up wearing a bra. Sometimes she tells me I am too thin and when she does I can hear that man Guy guffawing at the patent nonsense of it, just as he did that night in that restaurant, and though I love her to bits and would never wish her any harm, at moments like those I want to shake her.

If anything, my straggly hair and worn-out clothes and decidedly less than svelte figure are a childish reaction to her minding too much. I admire her minding, a minding which in her is more about self-respect than vacuous vanity, but when that minding is directed at me I rebel against it vehemently, ever the bolshy teenager. No, it is not for my mother that I want to be thin.

Friends then.

*   *   *

A few weeks ago I saw Mirry outside Tesco and wound down the window. 'I am so fat,' I shouted across the car park, first words I had spoken to her in a fortnight as we had both been away, and she laughed.

I met Mirry during lunch one day at primary school when we were five. It was across the long trestle table with its white and blue checked plastic cloth and over the perennial beetroot and salad cream and Spam. We asked each other our names and I said, 'Will you be my best friend?' It was simpler in those days. She has been ever since.

I can't think I am trying to be thin for her because she doesn't mind either way. In the past thirty-five or so years we have had exams and boyfriends, overdrafts and careers, sleepless nights and children, parties and political debates, and talked about a lot of things a fair deal, including diets. We have witnessed our respective weights shift a bit this way and that and discussed those shifts and forgotten about them. Most of the time, four pounds here or there we do not notice on each other, even when it is pointed up in no uncertain terms.

'I ate like a pig all weekend and put on nearly five pounds!' one of us might wail.

'Did you?' comes the invariable reply. 'Not so I had noticed.'

Sometimes we bemoan the fact that we are eating too much and that we have lost the knack of resistance, that in terms of eating less we are out of practice. For it is about practice. Then we might put on half a stone, even a whole one. Or if we are in the swing of things, we might take it off. It is within those normal boundaries that my half-sisters and cousins and colleagues and friends and I seem permanently to exist. Transatlantic telephone conversations with my half-sister in America more often than not include our eating and weight updates, admissions to each other as to where we are in the loop, comparisons, advice, condolences and what-the-hells. It is a constant cycle with us, as it is with all normal-abnormal women, infinitely banal and fascinating.

Our own fluctuations in weight are ever-absorbing; those in others might pass one by completely or give rise to anything from mild diversion to utter astonishment. The four pounds which on oneself make the difference between a waistband that is comfortably loose or breathlessly tight and can have a marked effect on one's mood for the week are quite lost on a friend. I can't see them if she grabs a handful of the said additional flesh and practically passes it to me. Seven pounds more or seven pounds less on someone else. If you notice them at all you might think, where did they come from, or, where did they go, are they hanging in a cupboard somewhere to be brought out again at a later date or abandoned for ever? Or you might think, half a stone, I could do with losing half a stone, and ask her how she did it. If she has lost or gained a slightly more substantial amount of weight you think, there is Mirry (or Martha or Char or Sophie or whoever) less ten pounds or plus ten pounds. Either way, she does not diminish. It doesn't make you see her differently. It doesn't make you think she is more or less attractive than she always was. It makes you think, there's Mirry, a bit fatter this week, or, there's Mirry, a bit thinner, and fatter does not mean worse nor does thinner mean better. The normal-abnormal margins are modest, they do not reach out to obese or skeletal extremes, so a bit fatter or thinner here or there is really just the same. That is my way of thinking about my friends, at any rate, and I presume it is pretty similar to the way my friends think about me and most friends think about each other, no?

I do not deny that there is competition between friends. With mine it is small-scale, humorous competition, none too serious, because it was years ago that we all accepted what we are and have just got on with it. Two will joke about who is going to be the first to fit into Gap size 0. That is a race I do not care to enter and I tell them they are daft, as if they didn't already know. Rachel becomes the proud owner of a pedometer which she got off the back of a packet of Special K and tells the rest of us she has done no fewer than 347,223 steps that day. We tell her in unison to hog off, we've done only twenty-two, and away she skips terribly happy. One of our number loses a load of weight – she wasn't ever fat in the first place – and we console ourselves. We are a bit wistful and tease her that she must have had liposuction and we wish we could look that thin, and in white jeans too. When we add that she looks great we really mean she looks great and flourishing but is still the same person we have known and loved all along.

In just the way that my friends' weight does not ever change my opinion of them, I recognise that my weight doesn't alter their view of me. They are my oldest, best friends, the coffin-bearers, as Sophie says. When my first son was born one of them came round and cleaned a hand-wash-only jumper that had been languishing at the bottom of the laundry basket for nine months and made me home-made custard, two gestures more memorable than any number of flowers. Her twin accepted no fewer than eleven telephone calls from me throughout the baby's first night home when Donovan and I were becoming increasingly hysterical and we hadn't a goddamn clue. I am just Candida to them, with my passive aggression, various cleaning obsessions (as I think is quite common in women with eating disorders past or

present – there are dusters and hoovers and a whole population of other such materials which travel round and round
my house in a permanent way) and a funny relationship with
lunch. As became evident during the wilderness years, they
care when I nudged too close to the wrong end of the
spectrum, was a miserable eleven stone or seven and lost
it a while, but the normal-abnormal in-between is a merry
topic over which to chew for the odd half-hour but not one to
spoil a good dinner.

I sometimes wonder if the people I want to be thin for boil
down to one or two particular friends as opposed to friends
in a more generic sense. I think of one who for some reason
has bothered me over the years, if less so now. She is the type
to shoot from the hip and speak her mind to all her friends.
She has never told me I am fat, but I think I have wanted to be
thin in her presence for fear of what she might be moved to
say if I am not careful. She has vitality, makes me laugh, has
saved me a fortune in psychoanalysis and I admire her
honesty, but it is an honesty that so far hasn't stretched as
far as fat. In matters of weight, I do not know a woman who
is completely honest with other women. Jesus, I'm not. I'm
full of shit. If a friend has put on weight and says so, I will
say, 'No you haven't,' when what I actually mean is, 'Yes you
have, but you still look like you only a bit fatter, what does it
matter?' While women acknowledge their own weight gain
to themselves and friends, they do not want it acknowledged
back to them by those same friends or anyone else. What they
seek from others merely is reassurance that they are still OK.
With this particular friend I have rarely scored the reassurance that others regularly give. To a, 'God, I'm so fat!' they
would all automatically bounce back with a nice, 'No you are

not!' – and that, though I never believed it, was oddly comforting. I always used to worry that this friend, unlike the rest, was a time-bomb. In her company I thought it was only a matter of moments before she, of all my friends, would come out with the excruciating, 'Yes, you are, very,' which I so dreaded and had spent so much of my life trying to elude.

I think of another friend in particular. She is over forty and has three children, has always been mega-thin and of a beauty that makes men weep. We were sitting on the grass last summer. I was in top-to-toe black, as usual had not dispensed with the opaque bodyshapers. She was in a Pucci-print bikini. This was something but something else was that, laughing, she started to do cartwheels. Cartwheels in her bikini. Then she did them some more, laughing all the while, and I stared at her abandon, for all the world that of a fuck-off teenager. I thought then, I don't want to be thin *for* her, I want to be thin *like* her. I want to embrace life and do the cartwheels-in-Pucci thing like she does. Then came the crabs and handstands and it was too much. I had to go inside and lie down for half an hour.

The curtains in the bedroom were closed although it was a sunny afternoon and I was not in the mood to open them. I stared up at the ceiling, at the joints and sinews of the old beams. A couple of tears darted into my ears which were bloody ticklish and annoying but they tripped a thought. The thought was that my cartwheeling friend is the type who gets angry and depressed sometimes with the best of us but she is also the type who lets go and enjoys the moment in a way I could only imagine. She is the type who not only does cartwheels in Pucci but moves to a part of the country miles away from all her beloved family, old friends and congeni-tally urban existence, for love and for the adventure of it.

211

Who has infinite children for regular sleepovers of madness and mayhem. Who goes with her husband and kids to Blackpool and consumes nothing but chips for three days on the trot, stays up all hours and has a ball. And so on. That is her way of embracing life. Meanwhile I think I could be like that if I lost a few pounds, but it's bollocks. It is making excuses and living on hold. Her way is about attitude and spirit, grabbing life by the balls and having fun. It is bugger all to do with being thin.

I lay there in the ineffectual darkness, the yellow-grey sombre made of sunlight through curtains, and thought maybe it was time not to feel envy but to sit up and take a few leaves.

Be thin for myself?

I have heard a lot of people say it is not for others, really, that they want to be thin but for themselves. Why? I want to eat chocolate, like vodka, enjoy the odd joint, stop cleaning and clock-watching, stay up till four. I want to appreciate the short time with my family and friends, to relish the fact I am doing the kind of work I like and stop wasting time caring so much about my bloody stomach. In short, do cartwheels *now*, not at some unspecified point in the future when I might have miserably managed to lose a bit of weight that I don't honestly need to lose. No, the kind of person who wastes a life trying to be thin, too thin, is not the kind of person I wish to be any more. I have become impatient and disillusioned. Of course it is privately pleasing not to have to shoehorn myself into an old pair of jeans; gently gratifying when they fit quite comfortably, when I manage to put off for another day the need to relent and buy a bigger pair. Being thin for my sake can give rise to those feelings as well as contribute to a more general self-respect but only marginally in proportion to the amount of head destruction the struggling to become thin tends to engender. It is not worth the candle and is not wherein proper self-respect lies. Proper self-respect is about knowing a few secrets in how to live life both realistically and for the moment. No, I do not want to be thin for me. For me, I want to forget about all that nonsense, throw caution to the wind, and get on with other things.

The day my father died on his seventy-second birthday of muscular dystrophy exacerbated by pneumonia was one of the best days of my life.

That sounds wrong. What I mean by it is the obvious cliché that it was a blessed release from his suffering and the event, while ostensibly sad, hailed a great achievement for a man who was supposed to have popped his clogs by the age of sixteen and a celebration of sorts for those who loved him. Throughout the day all the close family turned up at the mill in Oxfordshire, including Pop's brother, Pop's five children, his two grandchildren, son-in-law, two of his ex wives and one ex-wife's daughter by a subsequent and third marriage, as well as a jet stream of friends and nosy neighbours, former pushers, even a well-known chef bearing a welcome tureen. The dramatis personae that day was testimony to a chequered life led devoid of grudges.

A grey day. There was a single candle on the top of the chest of drawers in Pop's room, its still flame smooth in the gloomy light. Pop lay in his bed with a grey blanket covering all but his grey face. I had reached the age of thirty-four and had never known anyone I loved who had died. Never seen a dead body. It was smaller than when puffed up by breath and life; considerably shrunk. I put my hand on the wool of the blanket over his wrist because I did not want to feel his flesh no longer warm. At dusk I went into his room alone, candle by now straining to flicker with life, to tell him I loved him. We were always telling each other that. Even when not together we spoke on the telephone every day for over a decade and said it. So I was luckier than some who can't find the words till too late. But this time, confronted as I was by an uncharacteristic inertness on his part, I felt self-conscious and foolish; wondered if he was watching and raising his eyes to heaven at the cadence of my sentimentality.

The vigil was long and by turn hysterically funny and sad. We lolled about on the sofa and chairs in the sitting room, eating, drinking and gossiping, mainly about my sister's mottled love life. She had been talking about it to Pop almost up to the moment of his dying breath. When he did die she drew a short breath of her own, saw not much reason to stop and carried on amusing us and, who knows, him with her witty tales of woe just as he would have liked.

A year before Pop died Donovan and I moved from our flat to the house where we still live today. Four months before Pop died I gave birth to my first child.

Pregnancy had been something of a departure as far as my stomach was concerned. It had never throughout its varied history reached a state quite so huge. Fortunately its astonishing distension was a thing of intrigue for me as opposed to one which gave rise to hysteria. I stood side-on at my mirror and watched its hugely rounded shape for minutes at a time. It resembled not so much a water melon as a space-hopper, one of those inflated rubber balls on which toddlers boisterously bounce. I wondered at the skin's remarkable ability to

214

hold on to it and to stretch so without splitting, bursting open and making a terrible mess. I wondered at the baby's ability ever to get comfortable pressed up against my bladder, my lungs, my liver and lunch. The sight of the thin blue line seeping across its miniature white window and hailing my first child's existence had been in the flocked ladies' loo at a hotel wedding reception in Belfast. It followed a crab-stick dinner with which I had taken silent issue and was a sight that prompted ecstatic delirium. Soon afterwards, when I started to study graphic photographs of the foetus in pregnancy books, I could not picture a beloved son or daughter and did feel a momentary shudder at the thought of an alien squid taking up residence inside me which was gradually going to become the size of a deep-sea monster. Luckily, although I am squeamish to a degree, it was a feeling that vanished in a second. The corny side of me ensured that the excitement and miracle of what was going on in my troublesome abdomen precluded the major-league distress I might have otherwise experienced in the face of such a dramatic expansion. For the first time in my life there was a proper reason for a big – or very big, no, downright enormous – belly and it was not improper greed this time but something more than acceptable, infinitely wonderful.

Still, to keep any potential fat anxiety at bay I did take the precaution of never weighing myself throughout the forty weeks. I recognised that the scale's reading, distorted by exceptional circumstances, was never going to feel reassuring. The figure would invariably be higher than I was used to and, knowing me, in a blind panic I might lose sight of the cause and react unreasonably. Throughout, common sense and considerations at last for someone other than myself prevailed. I ate stably and healthily. There were a few occasions when I overdid it but then I knew about it: too much supper on top of the baby meant my lungs were squashed to the point where I became breathless even lying down and had to force into myself unpalatable quantities of chalky gloop to quench the fire of heartburn. By the end I guess I had put on a bit of weight that could not be accounted for by amniotic fluid, an enlarged womb and the baby, but after the birth, in the bullish shock of new motherhood, I forgot to care and the excess came off pretty sharpish and almost without my knowing.

Two more pregnancies, two more sons and seven years down the line, I am definitely thinner than my former normal. From the waist upwards even I can now see that I am not fat. My breasts used to come together roundly to form a cleavage. Breast-feeding has diminished them to such a degree that said cleavage is now the ethereal stuff of nostalgia and a bra – much to my mother's displeasure – has become an item with which I have dispensed as super-fluous. I have still never discovered a juicy vein running the length of each arm like those on my annoyingly sinewy friend, or biceps like hers, but I care less now because my arms have lost their chubbiness and do not spread against my sides like puffed wings. My cheeks have recently happened upon a little more definition than their usual sharon fruit, and if I tap my collarbone it makes a satisfying hollow sound like a builder hammering a bannister as opposed to that of a gloved hand patting an unsheared sheep. The historic pot-belly retains its perennial roundness but it is currently one of the smaller pots in the set. The thighs and bum are still sizeable but at least cellulite and stretch marks, I guess following a lifetime of non-virtuous temperance, are happily wanting. I do not walk the streets and into rooms feeling the freak that I used to and I can enter a shop knowing that there will be some clothes that will look fine; both things I daily appreciate.

I suspect reduction in size – a consistent stone and a half – is mainly the result of the fact that these days, while I still do not go in for any formal exercise, I do at least move, which is new. As someone who was married for most of my life to my bed and sofa and armchair, the sheer amount of physical activity involved in having children has been a revelation to me. In any given twenty-four hours, even if I do not manage to leave the confines of my own house, I feel I expend the energy of a long-distance runner. I probably run up and down the stairs a hundred and three times, to fetch a pair of socks here, wipe a bum there and tidy up everywhere. I lift three lively weights that jiggle and tug in my India-rubber arms and take all my strength not to drop. All the while I leap about the place urgently giving out glasses of water, cutting up bananas, getting in a stew about broccoli, wiping runny noses, struggling against kicks to score trousers on to legs, pulling on disobedient boots, power-walking to get to school on time, breaking up fights and kissing bumps better. It is their physical period and as such it is also mine.

The other day my oldest son said, 'Mama, have you got another baby in your tummy or are you just fat?' and I laughed.

Perhaps, I think to myself when I fancy dropping a few pounds, the fancying is on their account. I don't want to be the fat mother at the school gates who makes them feel ashamed. For I fear that for all my tactful monitoring aimed at eliminating fatism in my children, they are still appallingly fatist.

'Anyway, you're fat,' the disgruntled one of the moment will say to his brother witheringly.

There again, yesterday I gave another mother a kiss on the cheeks at the school gates to congratulate her on her good news. My sons were horrified and shrunk with embarrassment. 'Mama! How *could* you?' Tomorrow it will doubtless be some other solecism which I could not second-guess, such as my too-wide shoes, the way I say the 'o' in hello or too noisily scratch my ear. Being too fat would just be another one of many and it would be absurd to give in to it too seriously. You cannot insure against your children's random embarrassment. You would never leave the house.

Twelve years after meeting Donovan, eight years of happy marriage later, my father dead for seven years but on a good note, a trio of beloved children down the line and old friendships hitting anniversaries that can be counted in decades as well as years, I now see more clearly. Past relationships with family, friends and men, and the current, lasting ones, did and do not depend for their fate on my weight. I know that fine well. And yet, churlish abuse of my blessings as it may be, I still think that if I could lose a few pounds more then – well, then, what?

I put it off and put it off but then having written about half of this book I showed it to Donovan, who said it was one of the most depressing things he had read for a long time and that he had had no idea that his wife was so desperately unhappy.

He was shocked and upset. I was flabbergasted. He is an incisive critic who pulls no punches and does not go in for any English politeness or beating about the bush. That is why I am nervous about showing him stuff but so value his opinion. I had imagined he might tell me certain bits did not work here and various other sections needed more work there, and I had not expected praise. But this reaction I could not have anticipated for all the world. It was astounding and I was also very upset. Far from depressing, I had felt the tone of the book was reasonably positive, a bit like a confidence shared, even verging on quite merry. I had a good childhood considering its various upheavals – very fortunate in numerous ways – and I felt I had put that across. My current eating habits, while idiosyncratic, are pretty manageable and contained within a life no longer solitary but surrounded by close family and suffused with blessings. How could one of us have been so wrong?

I did not set out to write a book that was so autobiographical. I felt that I wanted to write about the wider experience of normal-abnormal women and, anyway, only the likes of politicians or other luminaries could rightfully go in for autobiography. Thus the book was originally conceived as a sort of memoir that mainly comprised reflections and observations that were much more general. I was reluctant to reveal too much of my own background. There are aspects of it which embarrass me, certain privileges which naturally incline me to feel I should shut up and put up. I did not want to upset anyone, least of all my mother who, despite adversity, has been a better mother than I will ever be. I am of the school that we too readily blame others for our shortcomings and did not wish descriptions of my parents to be seen as testimony for the prosecution. Other reasons were that I fear sounding self-important and do not like self-pity, and I worried that with too much of the personal I might fall into those traps hook, line and whole damn sinker. Finally, I felt quite sure there was not nearly enough in my memory with specific reference to food to fill a book.

So it was my very first draft took the form of an extended rant. Before long it became increasingly clear that a more definite structure was called for and more autobiography was the answer. I had to take the plunge.

The landscape of my past and my ways of thinking about things are so deep-rooted and familiar to me that I take them completely for granted. My childhood memories are the same set of memories I have had for twenty years; new ones seem to elude me. Who knows if the old ones are reliable. They are just there. The ways I control myself – not drinking; rarely taking drugs; having set systems with food; avoiding too many late nights on the trot; being so punctual; whirling around to keep my house unrealistically clean and tidy – are just me, routine. I recognise a certain absurdity about all of them but they cannot ever be surprising and do not really trouble me. Sometimes I feel a certain wistfulness when I witness in others unfettered joy and regret I have not let go more, allowed myself more fun, but Donovan feels much more strongly than that. On the evidence of Breakfast and Lunch, he feels I still have a serious problem.

Donovan has two brothers and no sisters. I have always teased him that for this reason he does not really understand women, the way they think and talk. Of course he knows the general gist of women and weight – that most favour the downward rather than the upward curve – but he could not be expected to be intimate with the detail of what goes on in the minds of a great many of them a lot of the time. Although I have been honest with him over the years and he has observed the petty neuroses of my day to day – just eating naked salad one night or bemoaning the fact I have gained a few pounds or eaten too much chocolate – I have not nailed him with the nitty-gritty of the tedious inner soundtrack which has been a permanent feature in my head but which is so much fainter now. I suppose I was careless not to antici-pate that that aspect of the book could have been surprising to him. But so very depressing? And I so very unhappy?

Deeply unsettled, I emailed a draft to Mirry. My best friend for thirty-five years, almost none of the ground I cover was new to her but she also said she was surprised I am still so exercised by food and weight; she thought I had largely overcome my anxieties. She did not go so far as depressing but she did tell me she found it sad.

I returned to the earlier sections. The childhood stuff I hope others might find affecting in some small way, vivid or interesting. For myself I think it is so much blah, blah, blah, been there, done that, no big deal. I reread the passages which distressed Donovan most, those concerning my morn-ing routine, my ways of eating in public and some of my other more questionable practices and beliefs. All those things were so familiar and entrenched that the gradual fading of them over the past ten years or so has been almost imperceptible. Looking at the narrative again with his reac-tion in mind, I realised that I was not actually writing about the immediate here and now but my distant and recent past, maybe up to the time I met him. In the face of such a reaction I have closely questioned myself. Do I still cling to walls and take measurements of every woman in every room? Am I to this day arranging the food on my plate with the precision of a stylist to disguise my greed?

The truth is I think I exaggerated or, rather, played a little freely with my use of the present tense. In fact I did not exaggerate, because I made none of it up. I lived by those various habits, practices and beliefs for a long time. They only receded very recently and have not been forgotten just like that. What I did was to make out that I am still living by them every day. Certainly they linger vividly enough in the mind for me to have described them in all their accurate detail. While I admit they do not malignly exist today as they once did, they have not entirely disintegrated. They are like dusty cassette tapes of music I once listened to again and again and again. Sometimes I take them out from the back of the cupboard, put them in an old player and press the 'play' button. I feel momentarily reassured, comforted even, by the sentiments and tunes, so familiar. I still like them but they bristle slightly. When I go back to them it is only fleetingly and not wholeheartedly. So the things I wrote that smacked to Donovan of a wife in turmoil remain relevant and valid for inclusion in the book, but it is new music I want to listen to now. A good life, with a husband and children, a solid roof over my head and work I enjoy have slowly stepped in dramatically to reduce the effect those old songs have on me. Other more vital preoccupations have necessarily come to the fore: the political – the hell of a Bush world – and, even more immediately, the personal. Shall we move to the country or stay in the city? What schools will our children go to and what is best for them? The most beneficial balance of work and motherhood? Motherhood, full-stop: so many mistakes already, how to put them right? How to curb my impatience and better show them how much I love them? Longing for another and at the same time not – too old, too tired and yet to win the lottery. Granny dying. Our parents getting older. Menopause and our own old age oddly looming. Sometimes, along the way, Donovan has lifted his eyes to the heavens when I eschew steak for supper and go for a salad instead, or been pissed off at the one time in five I eat mango at lunch instead of roast chicken with everyone else, having had too much supper the night before. It is certainly something which has raised its head in our marriage. He is largely sympathetic and understanding and accepting of my ways, but there were times, early days, when I was more like I described earlier in the book and he became exasperated. Then he said occasionally, 'We've got to get your eating sorted out. Why can't you just eat, what the hell does it *matter* if you put on some weight? Life's too short!'

He has not said that recently. I am less obsessed, less extreme. Or he had said nothing for a long time, till he read the book. It brought it all up again but he must be forgiven his reaction, for I was mistaken in the impression I gave. Today, while some old beliefs malinger like generations of bored, slightly menacing youths on the same street corner, other things are not strictly as I wrote.

One hardy perennial is the refusal to accept it when friends tell me I am thin. To my mind the compliment is comparative merely. At best they are telling me that I am thinner than I was when they last saw me (the implication of which, as I have said before, is not so much that I am thin as just less fat, an underhand insult); at worst they are just telling me what they know I want to hear, lying effectively. They never mean I am thin on the general scale of women's thinness. I want to say, what on earth are you on about? Use your eyes for fuck's sake. Look at Kate and Daisy and Anna and Sophie. They are what I call thin. How the hell can you measure me in with them? I am not a thin person, same way as I am not a violent one; never have been, probably never will be.

But at least today there is an element of contradiction in

my head. Today I also hear a voice which says that my weight and BMI are healthy and respectable. In the wider scheme of things I may not be actively skinny but I am within the realms of normal, and my neck and chest and arms are erring on the side of thin, not fat. I accept that.

Even so, I never intended to reveal my weight in this book. My weight had always come under the jurisdiction of the Official Secrets Act. So it was I resisted mentioning its specifics until Mirry read the first draft and told me it was essential. To omit it, she said, would undermine every word I wrote. I did not want to hear that, and itemising my stones and pounds over the years took more doing than some of the denser text, the fear palpable for several days. But now that I have laid myself on the line I even own that there are a lot of women out there who will look at the chart, see the nine stone this and eight stone that, and feel I have no right to call myself fat, to share the anxieties of those with a higher score, those who are genuinely overweight. What right have I, who on good days is a size 8?

Indeed, what right have I? Even at nine stone three – as I was till a few days ago and will be again – who am I to talk?

And yet I didn't make this book up. I hope most readers will recognise that and feel that the sentiments are entirely genuine, regardless of the scales. Still, the thought of some women reading it who are heavier than me and who might understandably feel angry and resentful has been levelling. Guy's words in that restaurant are not forgotten but for the most part I say to myself, oh for God's sake, get over it.

I weigh myself most mornings and for the most part a few minutes later forget the reading, don't really care. I can now pile my plate high as I like and find it funny, well, kind of, if someone thinks it impressive. True, I still do not eat breakfast and tend to go in for a lunch more modest than piggy. But when I nibble the ends of my sons' leftover sausages or eat a stack of chocolate as I do most nights I think 'yum' and just damn well go with the flow.

Last year was the twenty-fifth anniversary of the publication of *The Great Chefs of France*, my father's tome featuring the *foie gras* hedgehogs. The arm of the Muscular Dystrophy Campaign called the Q Trust – set up in his name after his death – had the idea of persuading ten or so leading chefs with the Academy of Culinary Arts to get together to cook a five-course dinner for four hundred and fifty people at the Savoy Hotel in London. It was both to celebrate the book, which in chefly circles has become something of a classic, and to raise money for research into the disease which killed Pop and continues mercilessly to beleaguer many others. Old masters – including Albert Roux and Raymond Blanc – and new ones alike collaborated to concoct a feast featuring recipes in the book.

The event was almost a year in the planning and I joined in. I had never been involved in anything like it before but it meant a lot to me that it should be a success. I wanted to contribute in any way I could because the cause was an excellent one and I remembered so fondly the making of the book. On his return from his gastronomic trips to France Pop had regaled the family with amazing anecdotes. His descriptions of what he had eaten, and the photographs of the various chefs and dishes, constituted my vicarious introduction to food of a different order from that of shepherd's pie and treacle tarts. I was fourteen and rather into hamburgers when he gave me a gleaming finished copy. It represented enormous toil and not a little merriment on his part, as well as a swift education on mine. I still have it, treasured if battered, with Pop's inscription: 'To Candida – in the hope that one day she will like some sauce other than tomato ketchup.' It is a book which represents my father's love of food, wine, travel, humour and determination to overcome adversity (the book was a bugger to produce; endless authorial and technical problems); in short, his admirable zest for life.

For several months before the big dinner I and about fifteen others went to meetings in the boardrooms and dining rooms of Claridge's and the Savoy to discuss details and join in tastings. I was extremely excited and enjoyed the whole process, not least the excuse to skive off from my solitary toil at the computer and the odd arsenic hour with my children. (The arsenic hour is five till seven-thirty in the evening, that oft-fraught window which incorporates the blood-sugar ululations of tea, bath and bedtime.) There was nothing I liked more than going into the West End to sit at a vast belinened table decorated with sharp pencils, headed paper, bottles of smart sparkling water and colourful fancies from the in-house patisserie, and making suggestions, debating the detailed arrangements and menu and giggling with grown-ups. I loved the unreal surroundings, the novelty of a fun but worthwhile project so divorced from my usual experience, the irresistible camaraderie of working with a team, the sense of common purpose and humour. The chefs always turned up in their whites, the rather put-upon little white buttons at their fronts endeavouring to restrain their stereotypical stomachs. Stomachs which competed for roundness and size, and which all in a row looked like a small galaxy of planets and made mine seem surprisingly modest.

'Oi there, Fat Man,' they would joke as a latecomer

arrived, a good chef joke relying very much for comic effect on the pot calling the kettle black. We all laughed, including the butt, though perhaps it was a joke I appreciated more than most because I had the added sense of relief that it wasn't directed at me.

At my wedding I had been on show in front of ninety of my closest family and friends. At the Q Trust dinner, on the other hand, I was going to have to stand up on stage before hundreds of strangers as well as close family and friends. My friend Hugh, who since he had cooked for Pop in France had written best-selling books on food and had several of his own television series, had agreed to give a speech. I was also lined up to say a few words. I did not want to let my late father down. I wanted to dress up (which I do very rarely indeed), buy new shoes and something significant to wear and even go to a hairdresser (something I had only ever done once in my whole adult life). The aim was to present my best front . . . and back and sides, and to do so meant not only writing a short speech that was not going to bore everyone to tears but also shedding about seven pounds. It is not abnormal, I don't think it is, to want to lose weight for a special occasion.

The dinner was at the beginning of February. Immediately after Christmas I embraced a regime of the usual no breakfast then fruit-only lunch; supper was salad with cottage cheese instead of dressing and three oatcakes, followed by yoghurt. I staved off hunger throughout the day by sipping my dread Diet Coke and popping my latest excellent discovery, the occasional sugar-free mint. I had little boxes of them all about me in coat pockets, in my handbag, in the drawer beneath my desk, the kitchen cupboard. Whenever the familiar portents threatened an aggressive chocolate takeover, I would place one of the white peppermint pips on my tongue to kid myself that I had just cleaned my teeth. Even at the tastings I took only one tiny sample from each of the proposed dishes, quickly followed by a definitive mint. I was very determined and by the morning of the big night I woke up feeling for me Surprisingly Thin. It was great.

I had been shopping in Bond Street with the friend who is a fashion editor at *Vogue* (we make an improbable pair, her in her Chloé, me in my catalogue). The last time she had taken me out was to look for a going-away dress for my wedding. We had gone to Valentino and Gucci but the prices had made me hyperventilate and, though we had a ball, I decided to 'go away' (down to the road from the reception to a hotel in the Banbury Road) in the same gear I had worn to go to the church. This time we went to Prada and I tried on a shocking pink (the black had sold out and my friend has a certain way about her that is almost immorally persuasive), satin, knee-length girly dress with no sleeves and an empire-line bow. With a *discount* it came to £850. In those hallowed surroundings and fitting into a size 8, I was so overcome with joy that I started making wild calculations and almost convinced myself it was, if not a bargain, then possible. It was not. The innate puritanism kicked in as is its wont. At the last minute I wavered and bottled out.

In the end I borrowed a black, sleeveless, satin 1930s vintage dress with a V-neck – rather more in keeping with my non-existent budget and my natural hue. Even the successful weight loss did not mean I could ditch a habit of over twenty years and go for a proper colour. It was ankle-length and cut on the bias. Any more than one piece of simple jewellery would have been a step too far but I did humour my mother with a modest paste necklace. And I squeezed my feet into unlikely high heels. My feet – the only part of me, Donovan says, only half-joking, that he does not love – are as good as deformed (though, oddly, I do not dislike them as much as I dislike my stomach). The arches are about as arched as a ciabatta loaf and I have bulbs of garlic for bunions. For this reason I live by one pair of shoes at a time and only buy new ones when that pair disintegrates. This is because whenever I do go shoe shopping I feel like one of the Ugly Sisters trying to force her monstrous member into the glass slipper. I somehow managed, though, to find a simple black suede pair which did not require surgery. My hair was salon-straight, not a tangle to be seen, and so clean and brushed and generally attended to that my whole head felt peculiarly light.

I spent the day in the bowels of the hotel sweating and laughing with the chefs. The manager let me have a room in which to have a bath and change. As the hour approached I was taking shots of Bach's Rescue Remedy at regular fifteen-minute intervals. It was a totter I made downstairs to the pre-dinner reception. My stomach had been flattened into submission by chocolate deprivation, measly mints and industrial-strength bodyshapers. I felt as though part of its lining had stretched up to my throat and clutched it. So I was uncharacteristically unmoved by the inimitable canapés and between animated conversation found myself, teetotaller that I may be, busily eyeing up the outsize bottle of vodka behind the bar.

Mirry, my supportive best friend of primary school provenance, was making sure people noticed how thin I had become because she knew that that would give me pleasure. When they pronounced me thin, for the first time in my life, I was able to believe them because for once my fingers could ride a bumpy course over the ribs in my chest rather than a smooth one. Tangible evidence. Under my dress, I knew my thighs were still a little roomy but, concealed under flowing black satin, I also knew that could remain my secret. Guy, the former lover who in a restaurant years before had elicited my misguided assertion that my figure might be all right if . . . but had not let me finish my sentence, was not his friendliest. This time I did not give a shit. Fred, who used to paint my picture, was generous with his compliments and cautioned, music to my novice's ears, that I must not get too thin. (Any such thing? *Definitely*.) Others commented fulsomely on the success of the evening and a cousin expressed astonishment at the reduction in my size. Meanwhile, Donovan's eyes expanded and sparked like rippled water in sunlight. It was the Pol Roger Rich, for sure, although I like to think that part of his looking upon me anew was not because the bones in my chest were showing (which anyway he does not find appealing) but because I had made an effort with myself for once, and *that* was a departure he could enjoy.

When we all eventually sat down at the forty or so glittering tables in the Savoy's lofty banqueting room (I don't think Pop would have allowed 'banqueting'), though I had been officially starving for some weeks, I felt not one jot hungry. The menu – *soupe aux truffes Elysées*; *escalope de saumon a l'oseille Troisgros*; *noisettes de chevreuil Saint-Hubert*; Vacherin Mont d'Or; *marjolaine, poires pochées et parfait à l'amande*; Savoy *café filtré* and petits fours – was all the stuff (though slightly adapted and updated to suit modern tastes) my father had raved about and I had wondered at back in 1978, and the committee and chefs and I had been discussing it for months, but now I merely picked at it. For that night only I was one of those people who had always puzzled me with their indifference to the food in hand. Although I passed it up, save a mouthful or two, I was not really indifferent. I had been closely involved with the long-term planning of it and throughout my diet I had told myself that I could eat the lot on the night; that was to be my reward for all the denial. But the moment came and the adrenaline had kicked in like speed. I was more interested in the shots of vodka Hugh had brought both us speakers from the bar. I have never understood how alcohol can take precedence over food, especially *such* food. I did that night, though, and it served me well. When I walked up on to the stage, approached the microphone and started to talk, I was not drunk but the nerves in me, mopped up by the electric soup as my father used to call it, were nowhere to be seen. At the end of it, all the chefs filed out of the kitchens for a toast and applause rent the air. The dinner raised a fortune for MD and was a triumph.

There is no denying that being thinner than my normal self for the night and in front of all those people felt good. I think the word some women like to use but I do not is empowerment. I do not seek to feel powerful – the notion does not interest me – and did not feel empowered. What losing weight did, more simply and less ambitiously, was to grant me a certain confidence and a few moments of quiet satisfaction. There again, was it the having lost weight or something else? I was among a lot of close family and loyal friends that night who were all remembering my father, eating fabulous food, drinking fantastic wine, rallying to the cause, embracing life. A lot of them, and even strangers, came up to me to say the evening had been brilliant. Not like your average stiff charity do, they said; it somehow retained a lightness of touch that was the spirit of your dad, full of vitality, informality, mischief and cheer. I felt a tremendous sense of belonging to a family and team who pulled off a certain achievement, however modest in wider terms, and felt part of something bigger than myself. In the course of it some happened to remark that I looked thin, others that I looked great. Being complimented on one's appearance of course bestows positive feelings of acceptance and pride that few can entirely dismiss, even those like me who on being flattered might be given to scepticism or defensiveness. But hearing that I was thin, and for once being able to believe it, did not turn out to be the apotheosis I had always sought. I just thought, that's nice, but does great mean thin; thin, great? The ones who said great might have said it because I had dressed up and brushed my hair, in which case the diet had been superfluous. The ones who said thin might have euphemistically meant gaunt and rather old, in which case, quick, pass us something wholesome even if it's not a *foie gras* hedgehog. Then I thought, touch of the corny notwithstanding, compared to the important things, really, what the hell does it matter?

The following morning, slight anticlimax though still buzzing, I got out of bed and automatically weighed myself. I had lost another pound or maybe stayed the same, even put one on, I cannot remember; but I do remember my first thoughts were, shit, how the hell do I keep the weight down now without a tangible occasion looming to work as an incentive? And, I am not enjoying this being thinner lark as much as all the effort to get here promised. It is a fleeting, superficial pleasure and my horror at being fat has simply been replaced by another scare: the thought of putting the weight back on and being fat again. Oh, please.

Taking it a bit easier than usual that morning, I sat back down on my bed and thought, now what? It is all very well being a rather unrealistic target weight and there is no denying that it – or whatever else it was – was great for a night, but whither? In normal life it would mean an infinite purgatory of lettuce leaves and cottage cheese and what would be the point when being thin (cosmetically thin as opposed to healthily so – the healthy margins being much wider), while fleetingly cheering, is not all it is cracked up to be? I wondered then not *who* it was all for, this constant dieting and striving and worrying I have so long gone in for, – I still had not been able to work that one out – but *what*?

The enjoyment of the means if not the end. The numbers game of dieting. The daily counting of calories and ounces; the feathers of virtue, the coal lumps of guilt measured in pounds and ultimately the one no different from the other. A private goal each day, scored or missed. The satisfaction of control, of self pity at the lack of it. A small excuse for a little self-praise or a rap on the knuckles. Certainly something to occupy the mind, deflect it from boredom, general gaps in self-respect; an excuse to shirk greater slights or ills or shortfalls of expectation. To procrastinate. A romantic dance of false anticipation. A fettering of the more serious business of reality. Gripping. But as Donovan so rightly had it, depressing.

On Christmas Night last year, staying at my mother's house, we had just finished unwrapping presents by the fire, children going on all cylinders, and I came all over queer. I felt so tired.

Mum told me to go up to bed. She brought me a hot-water bottle. I shivered and sweated and shook. So far, touch wood, I have been the lucky type who is never ill. My head felt as if it had been clamped by an outsize nutcracker and my skull was just about to give way. I was coughing like a cannon and nausea swirled across the landscape of my body like a tornado. I was the colour of sky before lightning and felt the silvering of the saliva on my tongue hailing thunderous vomit, but I did not throw up. I tried to put my fingers down my throat but they could not go through with it. Perhaps because I have not managed to be sick once in over thirty years I think I must have lost the reflex. For five days, and then for another five, I lay in bed urged by the doctor to drink plenty of fluids and keep my strength up with milk-shake and soup, but the thought even of water made me retch anew and groan. It was pneumonia and during the course of it I lost half a stone.

In early January the telephone began ringing again and life started to return to normal. My sister in America and various friends rang to ask how Christmas had been and I told them. I milked it a bit and said I had felt as if I was going to die.

'But, anyway, you must have lost weight?' they asked.

'Oh yes. I couldn't eat for a week. Half a stone.'

'Well, it was worth it then, wasn't it? And there were the rest of us busily piling it on. Lucky you.'

Er, yes and no, I thought, but mainly no. Really, really no.

Nightcap

Apparently – I heard it on a television chat show – George Best's mother took up booze for the first time in her life at the age of forty and died just fourteen years later, of alcoholism.

I am forty and have of late been getting into the vodka in my own small way. But since hearing the fate of Mrs Best I am a touch wary of making up for lost time. In the past, very, very occasionally and to the consternation of those around me, I did pop the odd shot of Bailey's. I enjoyed the vulgarity of it; it is a drink which lacks a certain grace but it was really just a liquid way of having pudding. About once a year I also might have had an evening with tequila, Pimm's or vodka and a whale of a time though I never could quite acquire any of them as a habit. Recently I discovered there is a vanilla version of vodka and the other night I was given a capacious bottle of the stuff. Some friends came round and I went for it a little bit, plus a few Lind'or chocolates besides, only minus the justifications, concealments or guilt. It is one step at a time. Slowly, perhaps, I am learning to let go.

Mum says her mother was something of an alcoholic but, unlike Mrs Best, Granny lived to ninety-four and did not die of it. Perhaps she was just a heavy drinker. Her penchant for the bottle did not curtail her self-respect or relish of life as a serious dependency on alcohol is wont to do. Every day in the old people's home where she lived for her last eight years, she dressed with the care of someone about to go to a smart social engagement, maybe luncheon as she called it in her favoured Chelsea followed by a few rounds of bridge; not institutional steak and kidney pie and peas with a whole lot of other half-blind, half-deaf old ladies. She wore silk shirts and pearls and patent leather shoes and brushed the organza of her mauve-grey hair. When my cousin took her husband to visit her, she quickly pulled her scarlet Chanel lipstick out of a shiny stiff handbag which had a loud gold clasp at its top and lived by her feet but never went far. She applied the lipstick as expertly as her arthritic, root-ginger hands would allow in order to be appropriately made-up in his presence, the presence of a *man*.

I admired Granny's enduring elegance and dignity in the face of general withering of the body and mind, including increasing deafness, gnarled joints, empurpled, diminished flesh and incontinence. A lot of people might have given up the elegant sartorial ghost by that stage but she had minded about physical appearance, her own and other people's, all her life. Although milky cataracts webbed across her eyes, she saw through them sharply enough to observe and comment upon the plainness or prettiness of a visitor, the more so if that visitor was related to her. Her weight was never especially interesting to her – she was much more exercised by clothes, make-up and hair – but that is not to say she did not give a damn. As she lay bedridden and dying last autumn, in moments of lucidity between trysts with the fairies, she gave up the ghost of elegance and appearance, of personal comments. Instead she stayed in her nightdresses, vividly remembered the 1920s, the parties and lovers, and had no truck with regret.

When I had an eating disorder, I often used to wish old age would come upon me sooner. I would will it to hurry up. Youth, with all its expectations and its desperate need to conform, was a burden which made me buckle. An imprisonment of sorts. Surely with age, I imagined, I would have done with all this pointless and wasteful anxiety about my weight, would have moved on and found the freedom to concentrate on other things. I yearned for the liberation that old age promised: it no longer mattering; my no longer caring about what I ate, food's consequences, what people thought of me and all else besides. But even as I became more normal-abnormal, and as my thirties neared their end, the low-key anxiety persisted and I wondered if I might not be lumbered with it into my fifties, sixties, seventies and beyond. I heard and read about and spoke to middle-aged and elderly women with eating disorders, and plenty more still trying to lose just a few pounds, battling against the years to keep their figures, whether or not they ever had one. And it depressed me. I thought if the constant awareness and dietary desires had not dimmed by their age, then whenever would they? Could I expect the mild affliction to be lifelong?

I am currently located somewhere quite central on the spectrum and am at least now lurching, inching, in the right direction, even if not expecting to near the golden crock of total indifference any time soon. And from where I am standing right this minute – I am with a large crowd of others – I believe the answer is yes. My companions and I will probably still be worrying a tiny, tiny bit, into our eighties. Even my grandmother, whose great boast was that she never noticed anything, noticed her own vague plumpness as she grew older. 'I was very thin when I was young,' she used to opine, even as a widow with great-grandchildren; kind of plaintive. She only stopped saying it when she hit ninety, forgot the pleasures of eating more than a sip of soup or teaspoon of ice cream and organically turned into skin and bone, without ever thinking about it, caring or trying.

I read an interview in a colour supplement with an attractive, slim, middle-aged, happily married mother who had a stunning job and house and husband. In it she said, 'If you met me you'd find it hard to believe that someone so outwardly calm and collected could harbour such a nasty, mean little voice in her head. It's a spoilt, churlish voice that says if I lost weight my near perfect life would somehow be more perfect still.'

That is a voice I hear in my head sometimes even now. It is one which in an ideal world I should like to discipline with common sense and family and friends all about me and work and fun and sometimes vanilla vodka. A voice which, if it cannot be entirely drowned out, I need to carry on urgently softening till it is one that is still and small and calm; I need to beat it into some acceptable form of submission before the Diet Coke dementia kicks in and does its lasting work for me.

As I was writing these last few pages, Carlo knocked on my study door. Carlo is Italian, about twenty-seven and handsome in a *Saturday Night Fever* sort of way. In the summer he wears cream-coloured jeans, no shirt and a gold medallion around his neck. He is a carpenter and whenever he comes to build another bookshelf for us is a cheerful presence round the house. He whistles and smiles and is full of shit but I like him and give him cups of tea and he flirts with us all, children included. Every au pair we have ever had has always fancied him like mad, all the on-a-permanent diet ones from Slovakia and the Czech Republic and South Africa; even the one called Barbara, a Belgian blonde bulimic who ate five bags of salad for supper then, after a pause full of silent conflict, five bars of chocolate. She stuck vast notes on her bedroom wall which said, '*Ne mange rien. Bois de l'eau,*' and beside a photograph of an erstwhile, thinner self in a bikini on a beach in St Tropez, another handwritten command in French: 'You fat pig, get thin like that again.' She was rather posh and sad and, we thought, a bit above herself for the likes of Carlo, but he had her in his thrall also.

'What you working at?' he grinned.

'A book,' I said.

'What's it about then?'

'Women and their relationship with food and weight. Me.'

'Oh, yeah? Kind of like, wanting to be skinny?'

'That's right.'

'A diet book? Oh, my girlfriend's writing a book about the same sort of thing.'

'Is she?'

'Yes, only a bit different in that she's really, really skinny, and there are all these books about how to lose weight, right, and not one about how to put it on! Can you believe that? It's doing her head in. Not one. That's why she has decided to write it herself. Do you think you could help her?'

'I would love to Carlo,' I say, slightly disingenuously. I would like to but don't know that I would love to. I own I have made progress, good progress; so far, though, there are limits to my empathy with someone who finds it hard to put weight *on*. 'I'm not sure I am quite the person, but if there is anything I can do–'

'I'll get her to call you, bella Candida. Ciao!'

And he is gone. My concentration rather shaken, my thoughts gradually but happily vere towards lunch.

ACKNOWLEDGEMENTS

Many thanks to Professor Steve Bloom, Professor
Janet Treasure, Louise Purbrick, Lesley Glaister,
Miranda Thomas, Agata Biernat, and Susan Hitch.
Also thanks to Antony Harwood, Rosemary
Davidson and Alexandra Pringle for their invaluable
suggestions and support and, of course, to
Donovan Wylie for his encouragement, belief
and more.

A NOTE ON THE AUTHOR

Candida Crewe has written several novels.
She lives in London with her husband
and three sons.